NVQs IN NURSING AND
RESIDENTIAL CARE HOMES

NVQs IN NURSING AND RESIDENTIAL CARE HOMES

Second edition

Linda Nazarko

MSc, BSc (Hons) Gerontology, RN

Blackwell
Science

Blackwell Science Ltd, a Blackwell Publishing company
Editorial Offices:
Blackwell Science Ltd, 9600 Garsington Road, Oxford OX4 2DQ, UK
  Tel: +44 (0)1865 776868
Blackwell Publishing Inc., 350 Main Street, Malden, MA 02148-5020, USA
  Tel: +1 781 388 8250
Blackwell Science Asia Pty, 550 Swanston Street, Carlton, Victoria 3053, Australia
  Tel: +61 (0)3 8359 1011

First published 1996 by Blackwell Science Ltd
Second edition published 2000
Reprinted 2002, 2004, 2005

Library of Congress Cataloging-in-Publication Data
Nazarko, Linda.
    NVQs in nursing and residential care homes\Linda Nazarko.—2nd ed.
      p. ; cm.
    Includes bibliographical references and index.
    ISBN 0-632-05225-2
    1. Nursing—Standards—Great Britain. 2. Vocational qualifications—Great Britain.
  3. National Vocational Qualifications (Great Britain) I. Title.
    [DNLM: 1. Nursing—standards. 2. Nursing Care—standards.
  3. Residential Facilities—standards.
  WY 16 N335n 2000]
  RT120.L64 N394 2000
  610.73'02'184—dc21

                                                                    99-059643

ISBN-10: 0-632-05225-2
ISBN-13: 978-0632-05225-7

A catalogue record for this title is available from the British Library

Set in 10/12pt Souvenir
by DP Photosetting, Aylesbury, Bucks
Printed and bound in India
by Multivista Global Ltd, Chennai, India

The publisher's policy is to use permanent paper from mills that operate a sustainable forestry policy, and which has been manufactured from pulp processed using acid-free and elementary chlorine-free practices. Furthermore, the publisher ensures that the text paper and cover board used have met acceptable environmental accreditation standards.

For further information on Blackwell Publishing, visit our website:
www.blackwellpublishing.com

Contents

Preface

I wrote the first edition of *NVQs in Nursing and Residential Care Homes* specifically for the 100,000 care assistants working in nursing and residential homes who are studying for NVQ level 2 qualifications. Since then I have had many letters from readers and have had the opportunity to meet many of you on my travels. Readers come from a range of backgrounds: many NVQ assessors use the book to work through the NVQ syllabus with students; care assistants who are not planning to study for NVQs, at least for now, use the book as a reference; and managers of nursing and residential homes buy the book and use it for training and teaching care assistants.

This book aims to supply care assistants and their managers with information and advice to help them meet the challenges of caring for older people in a rapidly changing environment. It provides an understanding of how older people feel about homes; an understanding of how age affects the body and mind; information on how illness affects older people's abilities; and ways in which staff can work to help older people enjoy life. It offers basic information about older people's legal rights, and it supplies details of information and resources available. It also provides guidance on good practice within registered homes.

This is an exciting time for care assistants working in nursing and residential homes.

At the time of writing the government is in the process of introducing the Care Standards Bill. This will change the way homes are inspected and regulated and will place more emphasis on quality care and the education and training that staff require to deliver quality care. The Care Standards Bill is expected to enter the statute books in summer 2000 but it may not be enacted until April 2002. When it is enacted the Registered Homes Act, that currently governs nursing and residential homes in England and Wales, will be repealed and homes will work to the new legislation. The legislation in Wales is expected to differ slightly from that in England. Scotland is in the process of developing its own legislation and standards. Northern Ireland will also develop its own legislation. Under proposed legislation all homes will be referred to as care homes, although it is expected that some will be known as nursing care homes, nursing and residential care homes and residential care homes. In this book they are referred to as nursing homes and residential homes, for simplicity.

In recent years, the number of older people cared for in homes has risen enormously and has now reached over a million. The growth in the numbers of old people in the population, changes in the health service, and the introduction of the Community Care Act have meant that people living in homes require higher levels of care than ever before. Since the mid-1980s homes have changed beyond all recognition. Standards have risen; now most homes offer single or double rooms that are carpeted and furnished to higher standards than before. Facilities that were once viewed as luxuries are now becoming standard. Older people, their families, social services departments, and health authorities now expect higher standards of care from staff. At the same time the people cared for in homes require more help with the activities of daily living than ever before.

The role of care assistants has changed dramatically. Many experienced care assistants have undertaken training within the home, attended study days, and spent time visiting clinics and observing specialists at work. Until recently, these achievements were not always recognised. The introduction of National Vocational Qualifications (NVQs) enables care assistants, for the first time, to gain a qualification that demonstrates to employers their level of skills.

Care assistants studying for NVQ qualification work through a closely monitored programme, which increases their level of knowledge and enables them to gain credit for practical skills. NVQ qualifications enable care assistants to increase this knowledge and build on their existing skills.

Care assistants, even those with years of practical experience, learn a great deal when gaining NVQ qualifications. This enables them to understand the problems older people face and equips them with the skills required to care for older people sensitively. This is good news for older people in homes, who benefit from higher quality care.

NVQ qualifications are gaining increasing recognition. The new government white paper on social services and the Care Standards Bill going through Parliament at the time of writing, demonstrate this. As part of this process, proposed new quality standards for nursing and residential homes have been drawn up. These standards, known as national required standards, are part of a consultation paper called *Fit for the Future*. The government will respond to the consultation for this paper in summer 2000.

These proposed standards specify that 50% of staff employed in nursing and residential homes must have an NVQ level 2 qualification. The standards propose that people managing residential homes must have a nursing or an NVQ level 4 qualification in management.

Employers recognise the contribution that NVQ qualified staff make to the quality of care and are supporting and rewarding staff who attain such qualifications. If the proposals are ratified then staff with NVQ qualifications will be sought after and doubtless paid more than care assistants who lack NVQ qualifications.

Universities and colleges of further education value NVQs. Students who attain NVQ level two and three qualifications are now able to enter university and train to be a registered nurse. The government is now proposing to develop an NVQ level 3+ qualification that would enable people to enter the second of the three year registered nurse education programme.

NVQs give many people who did not have the opportunity to do further training when they left school the chance to gain recognition for their experience. This helps build confidence and enhances the quality of care.

The quality of care is dependent on the skills of staff in nursing and residential homes. Older people have the same feelings, fears, and hopes as all adults. The aim of this book is to give you the information you need to help you understand older people and provide the best possible care.

The future for NVQ students has never been brighter. I hope that you enjoy this book and find it fulfils its aims. The feedback you have provided has been very helpful. I have done my best to use it to improve the second edition. If you have any comments to make please get in touch.

Linda Nazarko
E-mail: nursinghome.uk@virgin.net

Acknowledgements

Producing this book would not have been possible without the co-operation and help of many people. I would like to thank my former colleagues and the residents of Purley View who posed for the photographs in this book, my husband Ed who took most of the photographs, and Grahame Jones who produced the illustrations.

I would also like to thank the following companies who provided photographs and illustrations:

The Coloplast Foundation: Fig. 13.14; Arjo: Figs 10.3, 10.4, 10.5, 10.6, 12.1, 12.2, 12.3, 13.4 & 13.15; Kirton Healthcare: Figs 3.1(a) & 3.1(b); Huntleigh Healthcare: Figs 11.5, 11.6, 11.7, 11.8, 11.9, 11.10, 11.11, 11.12, 11.13 & 11.14; Parker Baths: Fig. 12.4 and Springhill nursing home: Fig. 6.3, and Convatec.

Thanks to all those at Blackwell Science involved in this and the first edition, for their meticulous editing and helpful suggestions.

And last, but not least, thanks to Rachael and Sam Nazarko, my children.

Dedication

With love to my husband whose enthusiasm
and encouragement helped turn a fireside chat into a book.

Thanks Ed

How to Use This Book

NVQs are National Vocational Qualifications. NVQs were introduced in 1988 and aimed to allow workers to gain recognition for the skills that they gained through experience. Ten years later, in 1998, changes were made to the NVQ syllabus. The paperwork that students must complete has been streamlined.

You must complete nine units from the NVQ syllabus to obtain an NVQ level 2 qualification. An NVQ consists of compulsory and optional units. The NVQ level 2 in care consists of four compulsory units.

Students can choose a further five optional units. The optional units are divided into two groups, option group A and option group B. Students must choose at least three units from option group A. The other two units can be chosen from group A or B.

Each unit is divided into elements. Each element has a number of components:

- The title – this describes the task
- Performance criteria – this describes how the task or work should be carried out
- Range – this details situations where you are required to demonstrate your skills
- Knowledge – this outlines the level of knowledge you require to carry out the task or work effectively.
- Evidence requirements – these requirements describe ways to gather evidence to demonstrate competence.

Reading this book as a whole will enable you to gain a greater understanding about the physical and psychological aspects of ageing. Each chapter relates to parts of the NVQ level 2 course. Students studying for a particular unit will find most of the information on that subject in a particular chapter of the book.

A list of units/elements and the relevant chapters is given here.

Description of unit/element	Name	Content	Chapter
Core/mandatory	O1	Foster people's equality, diversity and rights	1
Core/mandatory	O1.1	Foster people's rights and responsibilities	1
Core/mandatory	O1.2	Foster equality and diversity of people	1
Core/mandatory	O1.3	Maintain the confidentiality of information	1
Core/mandatory	CL1	Promote effective communication and relationships	2
Core/mandatory	CL1.1	Develop relationships with people which value them as individuals	2
Core/mandatory	CL1.2	Establish and maintain effective communication with people	2
Option group A	CL2	Promote communication where there are communication differences	2
Option group A	CL2.1	Determine the nature and scope of communication differences	2
Option group A	CL2.2	Contribute to effective communication where there are communication differences	2
Option group B	CL5	Promote communication with those who do not have a recognised language format	2
Option group B	CL5.1	Determine the ways in which individuals who do not use a recognised language format are communicating	2
Option group B	CL5.2	Develop and maintain relationships with people who do not use a recognised language format	2
Core/mandatory	CU1	Promote, monitor and maintain health, safety and security within the workplace	3
Core/mandatory	CU1.1	Monitor and maintain the safety and security of the work environment	3
Core/mandatory	CU1.2	Promote standards of health and safety in working practice	3
Core/mandatory	CU1.3	Minimise the risks arising from health emergencies	3
Core/mandatory	Z1	Contribute to the protection of individuals from abuse	4
Core/mandatory	Z1.1	Contribute to minimising the level of abuse in care environments	4
Core/mandatory	Z1.2	Minimise the effects of abusive behaviour	4

Description of unit/element	Name	Content	Chapter
Core/mandatory	Z1.3	Contribute to monitoring individuals who are at risk of abuse	4
Option group A	CU5	Receive, transmit, store and retrieve information	5
Option group A	CU5.1	Receive and transmit information	5
Option group A	CU5.2	Store and retrieve records	5
Option group A	NC12	Enable clients to eat and drink	6
Option group A	NC12.1	Help clients to get ready for eating and drinking	6
Option group A	NC12.2	Help clients to consume food and drink	6
Option group B	NC13	Prepare food and drink for clients	6
Option group B	NC13.1	Enable clients to choose food and drink	6
Option group B	NC13.2	Prepare and serve food and drink to clients	6
Option group A	W2	Contribute to the ongoing support of clients and others who are significant to them	7
Option group A	W2.1	Enable clients to maintain their interests, identity and emotional wellbeing whilst receiving a care service	7
Option group A	W2.2	Enable clients to maintain contact with those who are significant to them	7
Option group A	W2.3	Support those who are significant to the client during visits	7
Option group A	W2.4	Enable carers to support clients	7
Option group B	W8	Enable individuals to maintain contact in potentially isolating situations	7
Option group B	W8.1	Support individuals in maintaining social contact	7
Option group B	W8.2	Obtain specific information and literature for individuals	7
Option group B	Z13	Enable clients to participate in recreation and leisure activities	7
Option group B	Z13.1	Encourage clients to plan recreation and leisure activities	7
Option group B	Z13.2	Support clients during recreation and leisure activities	7
Option group A	W3	Support individuals experiencing a change in their care requirements and provision	8
Option group A	W3.1	Enable clients to prepare for and transfer to different care requirements	8

Description of unit/element	Name	Content	Chapter
Option group A	W3.2	Enable individuals to become familiar with new care environments	8
Option group A	Z6	Enable clients to maintain and improve their mobility through exercise and the use of mobility appliances	9
Option group A	Z6.1	Enable clients to exercise	9
Option group A	Z6.2	Assist clients to use mobility appliances	9
Option group B	Z5	Enable clients to maintain their mobility and make journeys and visits	9
Option group B	Z5.1	Enable clients to maintain their mobility in their immediate environment	9
Option group B	Z5.2	Assist clients with their preparations for a journey or visit	9
Option group B	Z5.3	Accompany clients on journeys or visits	9
Option group A	Z7	Contribute to the movement and handling of individuals to maximise their physical comfort	10
Option group A	Z7.1	Prepare individuals and environment for moving and handling	10
Option group A	Z7.2	Assist individuals to move from one position to another	10
Option group A	Z7.3	Assist individuals to prevent and minimise the adverse effects of pressure	11
Option group A	Z9	Enable clients to maintain their personal hygiene and appearance	12
Option group A	Z9.1	Enable clients to maintain their personal cleanliness	12
Option group A	Z9.2	Support clients in personal grooming and dressing	12
Option group A	Z11	Enable clients to access and use toilet facilities	13
Option group A	Z11.1	Enable clients to access toilet facilities	13
Option group A	Z11.2	Assist clients to use toilet facilities	13
Option group A	Z11.3	Collect and dispose of client's body waste	13

Chapter 1

Older People, Equality, Diversity and Rights

Introduction

This chapter provides information on the core units O1, O1.1, O1.2 and O1.3 – 'foster people's equality, diversity and rights'.

This chapter examines and discusses:

- Older people's role in society
- The legal rights of the older person living in a home
- The rights to health care and services
- The right to be treated with dignity and respect; dignity and respect are so important that the whole book contains material on this issue
- Confidentiality – discussed in greater detail in Chapters 7 and 8
- The rights of older people to make choices about how they choose to lead their lives; choice is one of the most important issues in caring for older people so this issue will recur throughout the book
- Information to help the carer provide care appropriate to the older person's cultural background
- Details of how care assistants can help people continue to attend church and practise their religion

---

Older people and society

In the past, it was unusual for people to live as long as they do now. At the beginning of the century when old age pensions were introduced few older people lived long enough to collect their pensions. During this century improved living conditions and improved medical care have resulted in people living longer than before (Fig. 1.1).

As you can see in Fig. 1.1, the number of people over the age of 85 will have risen from 70,000 at the beginning of the century to 1.2 million by the end of the century. Most people living in homes are women. Statistics show that for every 77 women over the age of 85 years there are 23 men. Statistics also show

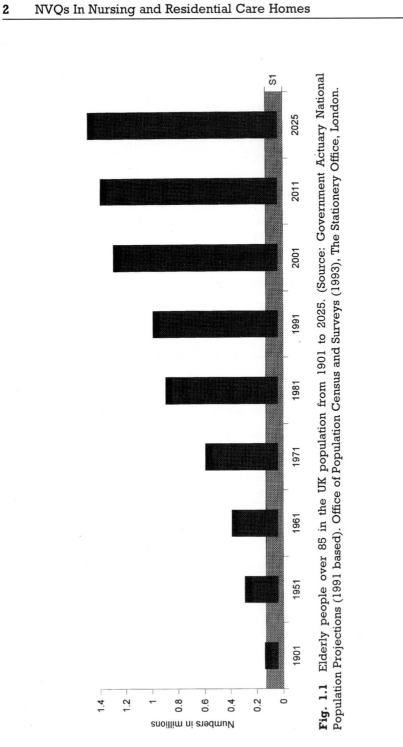

Fig. 1.1 Elderly people over 85 in the UK population from 1901 to 2025. (Source: Government Actuary National Population Projections (1991 based). Office of Population Census and Surveys (1993), The Stationery Office, London.

that older men are less likely to be admitted to homes than women are. When men are admitted to homes, they require much greater levels of care than women. There are several reasons for this. Women in the past tended to marry men who were on average five years older. When these men become ill and require care, their wives care for them for as long as possible. Research shows that these younger wives are well organised and obtain help from family members, district nurses and social services. The married older man is cared for at home for as long as possible. It is only when the older man's wife can no longer cope that he is admitted to care. Women still live on average five years longer than men and by the age of 70 two-thirds of all women are widowed or divorced. Half of the women over the age of 60 either had no children or have lived longer than their children. So women, because they live longer and married older men, are less likely to have anyone to care for them when they require help.

Older people and their families

We often hear people complaining that families no longer care for old people in the way that they did in the past. In fact, fewer families cared for older people in the past because there were fewer older people. At the beginning of the century, families often lived under the same roof. The family might consist of grandparents, parents, and children. In many cases, the family did not live together out of choice but because they could not afford separate homes. As people have become more prosperous, it has become rare for several generations to live under the same roof.

Research, though, shows that families still care for the older members of the family. This research confirms what many people often forget: older people have more experience and offer younger members of the family advice and support, while younger members of the family help with physical tasks which the older person may now find difficult.

There are seven million carers in the UK. Many have given up their own well-paid jobs to care for a member of their family.

Research shows that families do provide practical help and support for older people. Care assistants can help families remain involved when the person is admitted to a home; further details are given in Chapters 7 and 8. Some older people do not have any family and because they may not have help and support they are more likely to be admitted to homes.

The legal rights of a person living in a home

A person living in a home has the same legal rights as any other citizen. In the USA, there is a written constitution and every citizen is aware of his or her rights because these are written down. People being cared for in hospitals and homes have a series of basic rights that are legally binding. In the UK our legal system is older and has evolved over more than a thousand years. There is no legal declaration of each citizen's rights, but instead a series of Acts of Parliament and common law that define a person's rights.

People living in homes have not given up any of their rights when they enter the home. If the person wishes to leave the home, staff cannot forcibly detain the person except in special circumstances. If the person is at serious risk of injuring themselves or others then a doctor, social worker or police officer can exercise special powers to detain the person for a limited period. If this is the case, the person will be transferred to hospital or a specialist home for care by nurses specialising in caring for people with mental health needs. Consent must be obtained before care is carried out or medication is given. Forcing a person to bath against their will or forcing a person to take medication or have treatment is an offence. Sensitive care will involve working with the older person to meet needs, not imposing a regime on the individual.

Rights to health care and services

People living in residential and nursing homes have the same rights to health care as people living in their own homes. Older people have the same right to choose their own general practitioner (GP) as other adults. Most homes have a GP who visits on a regular basis and provides care for many of the older people living in the home. If the older person lives locally, her GP can continue to visit and offer medical care. Unfortunately, many older people admitted to homes are no longer in the area where their GP has agreed to provide care.

Right to medical services

GPs may be unable to care for people who have moved out of the area in which they practise because of the difficulty in travelling some distance to visit the older person in the home. In most homes, the older person moving out of the area to the home is asked if she wishes to receive medical care from the GP who visits the home. The person has the right to choose another GP in the local area if she wishes. In practice this can be difficult, as some GPs are reluctant to offer care to individuals living in homes. Some GPs state that older people living in homes require more care than older people living in their own homes, and they prefer not to offer this service. If an older person does not wish to have medical care provided by the home's GP, and a local GP cannot be found to offer care, then the older person, the family or the manager will have to contact the local Health Authority, who will find a GP in these circumstances.

Right to specialist nursing services

People living in homes have the same right to see nurse specialists as people living in their own homes. In some parts of the UK people living in homes receive excellent specialist care from nurses specialising in areas such as diabetes, continence promotion, wound care and stoma care. In other parts of the UK, the creation of National Health Trusts made it more difficult for some older people to obtain these services. Some NHS trusts introduced charges for such care. If the older person or the home was unable or unwilling to pay those charges, the person did not receive that care. Government then issued guidance that stated clearly that such charges are illegal. However, older people living in homes are considered a low priority by some NHS Community Trusts. Some nursing home staff have gone on special courses so that they can gain the specialist skills required to care for residents.

Right to therapy services

People living in homes are entitled to services such as chiropody and physiotherapy. Unfortunately, although the number of people living in homes has increased tenfold since the mid-1980s, the number of people employed to provide such services has not increased. In many areas staff working in homes find it difficult to obtain these services for patients. The local NHS trust has a responsibility to provide services for local people. If these services are not available, your manager can inform the local Community Health Council (CHC) which monitors the performance of NHS trusts and can make senior members of the trust aware of the problems. The telephone number of the CHC will be in the local telephone book.

Right to continence aids

People suffering from incontinence who live in residential homes are normally supplied with incontinence pads. These pads are paid for by the local NHS trusts. In most areas the district nurse visits and determines if pads are required. The nurse informs the NHS trusts and a certain number of pads are supplied for that person every month. If you work in a home run by social services, the pads will usually be delivered to the home. If you work in a residential home run by either a charity or a private concern, the pads will usually have to be collected. Pads are not supplied to people living in nursing homes. Here the pads must be purchased by the home and supplied to older people who require them. Homes that purchase pads for residents and people with continence problems must pay VAT on pads. The Association of Continence Advisers and the Women's Institute are campaigning to have this tax removed.

Right to confidentiality

When an older person enters a home, care assistants get to know the person's innermost secrets. You may, because of the nature of the caring relationship, know more about the person's thoughts and feelings than even the person's family. People who confide their secrets and share their feelings with care assistants do so because they trust care assistants completely. You must guard those secrets well and maintain the person's trust.

In some homes, and hospitals, sensitive information is bandied about. If a person suffers from diabetes this may be recorded on a label above the bed! In some homes charts giving details of the person's continence are displayed in corridors and lounge areas where other residents, relatives and even people delivering supplies can see them.

If the older person suffers from haemorrhoids (piles) she could be deeply embarrassed if staff mentioned this in front of another resident, even one who is sharing a room. Care assistants should be tactful and ensure that details of a personal nature are not discussed in front of others. This would not only be insensitive but also a breach of confidentiality. Confidentiality of information is dealt with in detail in Chapter 5.

Right to dignity and respect

All people have a right to be treated with dignity and respect. We all choose to work in a caring setting because we wish to care for people. Sometimes though something goes wrong and care assistants become insensitive to the person's need to be treated with dignity and respect. We have all heard of cases where people are placed on commodes in full view of others, or of cases where people are not dressed properly and care is poor.

Sometimes care assistants ask, 'What is acceptable and what isn't? How do I know if the care I am giving is good enough?' The answer to this is simple. If you would be happy to be treated in such a way, if you would be happy for your own mother to be treated in this way, then the care is acceptable. If you would not be happy to be treated as residents are treated, then the care is unacceptable.

Right to choose

Older people living in nursing and residential homes have the same rights to make choices as people living within their own homes. Unfortunately, it is much more difficult for people living within homes to exercise choice. People living in homes rely on staff to help them and many fear that if they complain they will be seen as 'trouble-makers' or 'moaners'. So many fit in and go along with the routine in the home. If older people do not make choices about how to lead their lives, they can quickly lose all sense of control over their own lives. They become disinterested in their surroundings, and physical and mental health deteriorates.

Research shows that in homes where staff work hard to enable older people to remain involved in decisions about their day to day life, staff and residents are more fulfilled. Regular meetings between residents and staff help older people remain involved. In some homes residents have formed residents' committees. These committees may plan recreational activities and in some homes they sit on panels to interview new members of staff.

Right to culturally sensitive care

We live in a multicultural society, yet few people from ethnic minority groups live in homes. There are thought to be two reasons for this. First, many people who came to this country to work are only now reaching the age when they may require care in homes. Second, care within homes is geared to the native population. Older people entering homes feel vulnerable and anxious. People who have difficulty in speaking English or who have a different diet or religion may feel terrified by the thought of entering a home. In some areas homes have been set up specially to cater for people from certain religious or ethnic groups. Special homes have been set up to meet the needs of people from Poland, Italy, Germany and Hong Kong. There are a number of homes that aim to care for people of different faiths. There are homes providing care for Sikhs, Jews, Muslims and people of other faiths.

From time to time, you may care for people from different cultures. If the person does not speak English, it can be difficult to communicate; further details on communication are given in Chapter 2. Care given should be appropriate to the person's needs. The person should, like all other residents, be treated in accordance with her culture and wishes. The diet should be appropriate to the person's culture; this is dealt with in detail in Chapter 6.

Right to worship

The person should be encouraged and helped to follow her chosen religion. People of different faiths celebrate special events. People of the Jewish faith celebrate the Passover. People of the Muslim faith celebrate Eid. People of the Hindu faith celebrate Diwali (the Hindu festival of light). People of different faiths should be encouraged to celebrate special festivals either with their family or with other patients in the home. With a little planning the home's calendar of celebrations can begin with New Year's Day and include St David's day, St Patrick's day, St George's day and all the other celebrations within a year.

Spiritual needs

People of all ages find that spirituality and religion play an important part in their lives. Many older people enjoy watching the Sunday service on television and appreciate the effort that staff have made to ensure that the minister visits. Many, though, would prefer, given a choice, to attend church. There is a great difference between listening to a service and taking part in one. Wherever possible the staff at the home should help older people who wish to attend church services to do so. The local ministers of religion can often put staff in touch with active church members who will escort the individual to church. Church members can befriend older people new to the area and help involve them in all types of church activities.

People who are not of the Christian faith also enjoy participating in religious services. Ministers and members of the Jewish, Muslim, Hindu and other faiths can help arrange transport so that, wherever possible, the person can attend religious services.

Conclusion

Older people have the same rights as anyone else to be treated with dignity and respect and in a way that is appropriate to their cultural background. Ensuring that people are treated in this way at all times is vitally important. Many homes have policies that emphasise and reinforce the importance of this.

Portfolio preparation

Your knowledge will be assessed in a number of ways. These include observation, verbal questioning and examining written evidence. You need to gather evidence that will demonstrate your understanding of how older people differ as much as younger people. You must demonstrate an awareness of the person's rights. You may wish to use the suggestions below to help you gather written evidence. Before beginning to prepare your portfolio, it is important to discuss this with your assessor.

- Many homes have a philosophy of care and this usually includes a statement about equality. Obtain a copy of this if your home has one. Prepare one or two sides of A4 sheets explaining how these aims are met within the home.
- Many homes also have an operations policy. This normally gives details of how the home is to be run in order to fulfil its stated aim or philosophy. Your assessor may want you to write a short passage on the difficulties staff face in putting such policies into practice and how you cope with these challenges.
- Check to see if your home has a policy on dignity and respect. Your assessor may want you to write a short passage on how this policy works in practice and how you cope with problems and enable residents to maintain dignity.
- If your home cares for people from differing cultural backgrounds your assessor may question you or ask you to write about how cultural and spiritual needs are met.

Further reading

Chester, R. & Smith, J. (1996) *Acts of Faith*. Counsel & Care, London. This book investigates how older people of all faiths draw comfort and support from their local church.

Counsel and Care (1992) *Not Such Private Places*. Counsel & Care, London. This book examines issues relating to privacy and dignity in nursing and residential homes.

Chapter 2

Communication and Relationships

Introduction

This chapter covers the core units CL1, CL1.1 and CL1.2 – 'promote effective communication and relationships'. It gives information about the option group A units CL2, CL2.1 and CL2.2 – 'promote communication with individuals where there are communication difficulties'. It provides information on option group B units CL5, CL5.1, CL5.2 – 'promote communication with those who do not use a recognised language format'. The material relating to each unit is clearly marked.

This chapter:

- Provides information and guidance to enable you to communicate effectively
- Explains how physical disabilities affect the cause of communication problems
- Discusses the particular problems facing stroke patients
- Explains the types of communication problems stroke patients face
- Outlines the problems people with Parkinson's disease face
- Discusses the different types of deafness
- Explains how to help older people use hearing aids
- Explains how confusion and dementia can cause communication problems
- Discusses ways of communicating with people who are unable to speak

---

The importance of effective communication

The ability to understand others and to make ourselves understood is a skill we often take for granted. In some circumstances, perhaps on holiday abroad, we have difficulty in communicating with others. Ending up with the wrong meal, being directed to the wrong place or being thought a little crazy by the locals is often part of the fun of being on holiday. Sometimes, though, difficulty in communication can be maddening.

Older people living in nursing and residential homes often have difficulty in understanding what care assistants are saying. If an older person does not understand what has been said then the reply can be inappropriate. You may think that the older person is confused. Some older people understand what the care assistant has said but have difficulty in making themselves understood.

Older people who have difficulty in understanding others or making themselves understood can react in different ways. Some can become frustrated, angry and aggressive, whilst others can become withdrawn and depressed. The ability to communicate is very important. Sometimes, because of illness, older people can have great difficulty in communicating their needs. Care assistants who are aware of the reasons why older people may have difficulty in communicating can use a range of skills to remove barriers that prevent communication.

Barriers to communicating with older people

Older people are admitted to nursing and residential homes because it is no longer possible to provide the care required at home. Most people living in nursing and residential homes are in their eighties and nineties. Most older people, even of this age, continue to live at home. Those who enter nursing and residential homes do so because they are too infirm to continue living at home. Some individuals are physically frail but very alert. Some are physically well but confused. Others are both physically and mentally frail. Most older people do not wish to leave their own homes and live in 'a home'. Older people admitted to homes often feel anxious and upset because of the move. They may become withdrawn and unwilling to communicate. Care assistants who spend time getting to know the person and encouraging the individual to express her feelings make an important contribution to her care.

Effective communication

Communication is not simply about the ability to speak and understand speech. We use all five senses to communicate and receive information:

- Visual – seeing
- Auditory – hearing

- Olfactory – smelling
- Kinaesthetic – feeling
- Gustatory – tasting

We receive input from all five senses. If you walk in the garden, your skin will sense temperature. Your vestibular system will sense whether the ground is uneven or not. Your olfactory system will allow you to enjoy the scent of the flowers and your auditory system will enable you to hear the birds sing. Your brain integrates all these sensory stimuli and you respond. If it is freezing cold, the garden is like a mud bath and the birds are dive bombing your washing, you will probably retreat indoors. If it is warm and pleasant, you will probably remain in the garden. You make these decisions because of information received from a fully functioning sensory system. Older people often have sensory difficulties that make communication difficult. The older person with poor vision will find it hard to see the expression on your face. She may think you are being serious when you are joking. The person with poor hearing may not hear the joke in your voice. The person with a poor sense of smell may not be aware of what is for lunch because, unlike you, she cannot smell the joint roasting.

Good communication is about finding out who the person is. It is about finding out what the person's values and hopes are. We do this in our everyday lives. When we meet people socially for the first time we ask gentle probing questions: 'What do you do?', 'Is Sam your only child?'. We probe gently to find out about the person. We make allowances for people and compensate gently for any limitations they have. Yet often in homes the staff do not really get to know the people they care for.

Communication within the home

Nursing and residential homes are busy places. Residents require more care than ever before and there is always something to do. Sometimes it can be difficult to make time to get to know people and to talk to them. Sometimes an individual relates better to some members of staff and those people really know the individual as a person; but the other staff do not.

The way work is organised within a home can make communication easy or difficult. Many homes have now introduced a key worker scheme. This means that the individual is looked after by a small number of people. Key worker schemes are popular with staff and residents. They help make care personal and help improve quality. Key worker schemes depend on effective communication. When communication is poor, the quality of care suffers.

Life histories

Some people living in homes work with their key worker or another member of staff to make a life history. Some individuals like to make a picture collage. This can include pictures of the person in different stages of life together with family, friends and loved ones. Others like to make a book about their life. You can buy a book, fill in details, and add pictures or make your own. Some people like to paint or create a tapestry.

Life histories give you information about a person and enable you to strike up a conversation and get to know the person.

Improving your communication skills

We communicate in a range of ways. The most powerful means of communication is non-verbal. You know exactly what mood your partner is in by the way he or she enters the house. A slammed car door, throwing off a coat and a rigid facial expression speak volumes.

Be aware of how residents will interpret your body language. Many people who find it difficult to communicate become very sensitive to body language. It is all very well saying that you have plenty of time but if you are standing up and glancing at the door every few minutes your body language is contradicting your words and residents *will* notice. You can use body language to reinforce your words. When you say you are unhurried, look unhurried. When you are listening look at the person, lean forward, use touch to reinforce your words.

How physical disabilities can affect the ability to communicate

Physical disabilities can affect the individual's ability to communicate in a number of ways. Strokes can affect the ability to understand speech and to speak. Parkinson's disease can cause individuals to have difficulty forming words, and speech can sound slurred. People who are deaf may be unable to hear clearly, even when wearing a hearing aid. Hearing aids amplify all sound and background noise can make it difficult to hear clearly. Hearing aids can also make speech sound distorted and so difficult to understand.

Communication and stroke

How strokes affect the ability to communicate

Imagine for a moment that you have had a stroke: you have no feeling in half of your body, you have difficulty understanding what is said, and it is difficult to explain what you mean. This is how stroke affects many of our residents. Stroke and the communication problems that often accompany it can make people want to curl up and die. Yet we can enable people to communicate after stroke if we understand the difficulties they face. Strokes can cause communication problems if they affect the speech centre in the brain. In some cases, older people do not understand what we are saying – it is as if we were speaking a foreign language. These people cannot receive and make sense of the messages we send them in our speech; this is known as receptive dysphasia.

There are degrees of dysphasia. People with mild dysphasia understand most of what is being said. Tiredness, background noise, people speaking too quickly or more than one person speaking at once affect their ability to understand. People with moderate dysphasia find it more difficult to follow conversations: long and complicated sentences are difficult to follow; some words are only partly understood. The individual may have difficulty concentrating and may be able to understand the start of a conversation but become confused if the conversation is too long. People with severe dysphasia may have difficulty in understanding even single words.

Many people who suffer from dysphasia after a stroke find that their condition gradually improves over weeks and months. People who are suffering from receptive dysphasia rely on tone of voice, movement, and gestures to help fill in the words that they do not understand. Care assistants should ensure that older people who need glasses are wearing them, as this will help the dysphasic person to 'hear' and communicate.

Some individuals understand every word and gesture but cannot find the right words to communicate. They mix up words and may say 'yes' instead of 'no' or 'plate' instead of 'cup'. Some individuals have difficulty in finding the correct word and use a similar word instead. This difficulty in finding the correct word is known as anomia and is part of a general difficulty in expressing what they want to say. This is known as expressive dysphasia.

Strokes can affect the muscles of the throat, tongue, lips, and face. Some older people have difficulty in swallowing after a stroke. Many older people wear dentures and these are kept in place partly by the muscles in the mouth. If these muscles are affected, dentures can slip around or be almost impossible to wear.

Poor muscle control and difficulty with dentures can make it difficult for individuals to form words. This difficulty in articulating is known as dysarthria.

Some individuals lose the ability to speak. This is known as aphasia.

Reading and writing

Strokes can affect the vision; often individuals can only see out of half of each eye, which makes it difficult to read. This is known as hemienopia. It is important that older people who have worn glasses before a stroke continue to wear glasses following the stroke. Strokes can change the vision and an eye test can be arranged to see if new glasses are required. Sometimes words make no sense to an individual; this may improve in the weeks and months after a stroke.

Strokes can paralyse limbs and can cause individuals to lose the ability to write. Some older people can learn to write with a non-affected hand. Speech and language therapists can assess individuals with such problems and can help them to regain skills.

How care assistants can help

It is important to realise that many people can recover most if not all speech following a stroke. Recovery is dependent on the severity of the stroke, therapy from speech therapists, the individual's motivation and the help and encouragement you offer. Care assistants can really make a difference and can help older people to recover or cope with communication problems after a stroke.

In many areas people who have suffered a stroke are invited to a 'stroke club'. These are normally held in local community health centres once or twice each week. The stroke club offers physiotherapy and exercise that help some stroke patients recover strength and movement to weakened or paralysed limbs. In other cases, exercise helps prevent deformity that often develops if paralysed limbs are not moved and exercised. Speech therapy is also offered, normally consisting of individual and group speech therapy. Many people who suffer from strokes begin to recover speech but are conscious that their speech sounds slurred and strange at first. Speaking to others with similar problems at a stroke club helps individuals gain confidence. Care assistants are often asked to escort older people to stroke clubs, and some are asked to remain with the individual during the session.

Golden rules to help stroke patients communicate

- Speak slowly
- Use simple clear language
- Use short sentences
- Only ask one question at a time
- Only give one piece of information at a time
- Use gestures
- Encourage the individual to use gestures
- Encourage the individual to speak
- Ensure that the individual who requires glasses is wearing them
- Ensure that the individual who requires a hearing aid is wearing it
- Listen and be patient

Further information

Action for Dysphasic Adults
1 Royal Street
London SE1 7LL
Tel 020 7261 9572
This is a charity that provides information to dysphasic people, their care assistants and professionals. It produces a number of booklets that are supplied free to professionals, care assistants and dysphasic people, including:

- *Lost for Words*, a general booklet about dysphasia
- *Stroke and Dysphasia*, a simple diagrammatic booklet
- *How to Help the Dysphasic Person* in the early stages, with comprehension and speech, with reading and writing, with total communication and complicating factors with dysphasia.

Parkinson's disease

Parkinson's disease is a disorder of the brain. Disorders affecting the brain are referred to as neurological diseases or disorders. Parkinson's disease is a progressive neurological disease. It is caused by a reduction in dopamine. Dopamine enables nerve cells to transmit messages to each other. An individual suffering from Parkinson's disease has difficulty in moving because of the disease. The disease also affects the ability to move the muscles in the mouth and tongue that are used to form words. Individuals suffering from Parkinson's disease often have difficulty in speaking clearly and their words can become slurred. The disease is now treated with a number of drugs that help replace the dopamine shortage that causes the disease. At first, the individual with Parkinson's disease appears to have fully recovered because of the medication. As the disease progresses, greater amounts of medication are required. Individuals in the early stages of Parkinson's disease are normally able to live at home. It is only in the later stages of the disease that they are admitted to nursing and residential homes.

At this stage, many older people suffering from Parkinson's disease are taking large amounts of two or more drugs to control the disease. These drugs work for shorter and shorter periods and in the final stages of the disease one of these drugs may be given as often as every three hours while the individual is awake.

Individuals who have Parkinson's disease may be able to speak clearly if they have recently had some medication but as the medication begins to wear off they may have great difficulty in forming words. Sometimes the drugs given to control Parkinson's disease can cause the individual to hallucinate or become confused.

Golden rules to help patients with Parkinson's disease communicate

- Speak slowly and clearly
- Give the individual time to speak
- Be aware that ability to speak will vary
- Be patient
- Check that you have understood what has been said
- Encourage the individual to speak

Further information

The Parkinson's Disease Society
United Scientific House
215 Vauxhall Bridge Road
London SW1V 1EJ
Tel. 020 7383 3513
The Parkinson's Disease Society produces a number of excellent booklets giving advice on communication and other aspects of Parkinson's Disease. You can obtain these by writing and enclosing a stamped self addressed envelope.

How deafness affects the individual's ability to communicate

Hearing loss is often referred to as the 'hidden handicap'. It is very common; approximately 7.5 million people in the UK have some degree of hearing loss. It is estimated that 4 million people would benefit from hearing aids but only 2.5 million actually have one. Hearing deteriorates as people age and by the age of 70, approximately 60% of people have hearing loss. This figure rises to 90% by the age of 90 years.

Most people living in nursing and residential homes are in their eighties and nineties and most of them will suffer from hearing loss. This affects their ability to understand and respond to care assistants and to others living in the home. Unfortunately, some people who meet deaf people automatically dismiss them as stupid. Older people with hearing loss state that others are inclined to 'talk over them' and that people who are deaf 'tend to be left out of conversations'. Other people are 'inclined to think that deaf people are not with it'.

Many older people with hearing loss find communicating with others extremely frustrating. If they feel that people are ignoring them, talking over them or treating them as though they were senile, they may simply give up trying to communicate. As one lady with hearing loss stated: 'If they make no effort why should I bother?' Care assistants who understand the causes and effects of deafness will be able to communicate more effectively with older people with hearing loss, and can encourage them to communicate and take part in the daily life of the home.

Causes of hearing loss

Wax

The commonest cause of hearing loss is wax in the ears. Even older people who suffer from deafness find that their hearing is improved if a build-up of wax in the ear is removed. Older people who appear to be deaf should have their ears checked by a doctor who will use an instrument known as an auroscope to check for the presence of wax in the ear.

Normally any wax in the ear is softened by putting drops in one or both ears three times daily for up to five days. Care assistants in residential homes may be asked to put these drops in an older person's ears. In nursing homes the ears are then normally syringed by a registered nurse; in residential homes, the district nurse may visit to syringe the ears.

Registered nurses often ask the care assistants to help with this procedure. The older person is seated in a chair and the procedure explained. Normally tap water is heated to body temperature (37°C) and drawn up in a metal syringe designed specially for syringing ears. The assistant places a plastic sheet and then a towel around the older person's shoulders and neck. The nurse squirts water from a syringe into the ear at an angle; the water trickles out of the ear and is caught in a kidney shaped dish by the assistant. The syringing washes the softened wax out of the ear and it is collected with the water in the dish. Many registered nurses now use an electric ear-syringing machine. The water is placed into a reservoir and is trickled into the ear using a special nozzle.

The doctor normally checks that the ears are clear of wax on the next visit to the home. If hearing is still not normal then the doctor will consider that the individual is suffering from hearing loss and will arrange a hearing test at the local hospital. Hearing tests are known as audiograms and cannot be carried out if ears are full of wax.

Conductive deafness

Conductive deafness is caused by damage or obstruction to the structure of the ear. Wax in the ear, by blocking the ear, can cause conductive deafness, and hearing is restored when the wax is removed. A heavy cold can cause the ears to become blocked and can cause temporary conductive deafness. An ear infection, which if untreated can persist for months or years, can cause conductive deafness. A perforated eardrum can cause deafness; a repair of the perforation can restore hearing.

Sensory neural deafness

Although sensory neural deafness is the most common in older people, there is no treatment available. As adults age the nerve that connects the ear to the brain, the auditory nerve, becomes less sensitive to noise, and the ability to hear is reduced. Hearing is lost first at higher frequencies. This means that older people with hearing difficulties can hear low-pitched noise quite well but have difficulty with higher pitched sounds. Women tend to speak at a higher pitch than men and many older people find it more difficult to follow a woman's speech than that of a man. The only available treatment for sensory neural deafness is to make sounds louder so that the individual can hear. Hearing aids are used to amplify sounds so that people with sensory neural deafness can hear.

Hearing aids

If an older person has difficulty hearing, their GP writes a letter to the ear, nose and throat specialist at the local hospital. The person visits the hospital as an outpatient and hearing is tested. The type of deafness and causes are identified. If the individual is suffering from sensory neural deafness, arrangements are normally made for a hearing aid to be supplied.

Hearing aids consist of two main parts. The earpiece, which is made of clear plastic, fits into the ear. Each ear piece is made especially for the individual. A mould of the ear is taken and the ear piece is made to fit snugly into the ear. A tube connects the ear piece to the amplifier section of the aid. The amplifier section is normally known as 'the body' of the aid. There are several different strengths of amplification to suit the level of deafness. The body is mass produced. Most older people who are supplied with NHS hearing aids are supplied with an aid that fits behind the ear. People who are extremely deaf may be supplied with a different type of aid that has an earpiece attached to a long cord. The body of the aid is the size of a pocket calculator and is clipped onto the chest over clothing.

Encouraging and helping older people to use their hearing aids

Many older people who have been supplied with hearing aids no longer use them. This is known as 'fruit bowl syndrome' because older people often leave their unused hearing aids in fruit bowls. In one survey of nursing and residential homes, half of the older people who had hearing aids did not wear them. The reasons given were that they found them difficult to put in and adjust or that the aids no longer worked.

Older people living in homes often find it difficult to perform tasks that require fine muscle control. They find it difficult to do up small buttons, and similar tasks. This may be because of illness. Arthritis can leave fingers stiff; Parkinson's disease can cause a tremor. In most cases, older people do not ask care assistants for help: 'they have enough to do'. Earpieces must be fitted firmly into the ear if the aid is to work. Aids must be turned on and put on the correct setting. The setting varies from individual to individual and environment to environment but is set at the level that enables the older person to hear easily. Batteries must be changed regularly. These simple tasks take only a few minutes but enable older people to communicate. This saves time spent *trying* to communicate and reduces frustration; it also makes a real difference to the person's quality of life.

Helping people with hearing aids to hear

Many people, including some registered nurses, think that if an older person has a hearing aid they can hear normally. Unfortunately, this is not the case. A hearing aid works by amplifying all sound and aids can easily distort hearing. Care assistants communicating with older people who have hearing loss, including those who wear hearing aids, should use special techniques to make it easier for individuals to understand them. These include:

- Cut down on background noise. Close the door if it is noisy outside. Close the window to reduce the roar of traffic.
- Move near to the person.
- Speak a little more loudly than usual – but do not shout. Shouting can appear threatening. It also distorts the voice, raising the pitch and making it more difficult for the person to hear.
- Always face the person.
- Speak directly to the person. Do not attempt to have conversations with more than one person at the same time. The deaf person will have difficulty following this.
- Do not cover your mouth whilst speaking.
- Speak slowly and clearly.
- If you have not been understood, rephrase the sentence using different words with similar meanings.
- Check that the individual has understood.
- Use gestures.
- Offer to write things down.

Communicating with deaf people who do not have hearing aids

Hearing aids can only help people who have some hearing. Some deaf people are totally deaf and are not helped by hearing aids. In this situation care assistants must find other ways to communicate. Many profoundly deaf older people have learnt to lip-read. Using the techniques above will enable people who lip-read to work out what you are saying.

Some older people do not have hearing aids because they are waiting for an appointment for one to be fitted. It can take six months to obtain an appointment to see the ear, nose and throat specialists at many hospitals. It can take a further three months to obtain a hearing aid. In these circumstances, the care assistant can write things down for the older person. It can be helpful to supply a notebook and pen, which the older person carries. You can then write down messages and the older person can reply. Remember to write clearly. If the person's eyesight is poor, writing in large letters can help.

Further information

The British Association of the Hard of Hearing (Hearing Concern)
7–11 Armstrong Road
London W3 7JL
Tel. 020 8743 1110
This organisation operates a scheme known as the sympathetic hearing scheme, which aims to make people more aware of hearing difficulties. The organisation produces leaflets, and a video that can be hired and enables you to understand what speech sounds like to hearing aid wearers. The association is run by people who are hard of hearing. It has a network of volunteers and may be able to provide a volunteer speaker to visit the nursing or residential home where you work, or your college, to speak to a group of care assistants. The association also produces a magazine four times a year.

The British Deaf Association (BDA)
1–3 Worship Street
London EC2A 2AB
Tel. 020 7588 3520
This is an organisation for deaf people. It produces a monthly newsletter as well as information sheets and leaflets.

The Royal National Institute for Deaf People (RNID)
19–23 Featherstone Street
London EC1Y 8SL
Tel. 020 7296 8000
The RNID produces a guide to local and national services for deaf people, plus a range of useful leaflets including *The Ear and How It Works* and *Understanding Hearing Aids*.

Communicating with older people suffering from confusion

Communicating with older people who suffer from confusion is perhaps one of the greatest challenges that care assistants face. It is difficult and some care assistants feel that it is not worth trying because they will be unable to 'get through' to the individual. Often a little time and patience will pay dividends and will enable you to communicate with the confused older person. This enables you to meet the person's needs. People who have their needs met are more likely to be relaxed, settled and happy within the home. It is important to be aware of the causes of confusion as this will affect how you can communicate with the individual.

Causes of confusion

There is always a reason for confusion. Sometimes staff assume that if someone becomes confused, 'It's just her age, what do you expect at 92'. There are two major causes of confusion: an acute illness, or the individual is suffering from a neurological disease such as senile dementia.

Older people who have suddenly become confused are usually ill. People who have a chest infection or a urine infection often become confused. Care assistants often know individual residents better than senior staff because they spend more time with them. They can often observe a cough or notice that an older person's urine smells. They should inform nursing staff, and nursing and medical staff should investigate and treat.

Medication can cause confusion. Care assistants, because they spend a great deal of time with residents, are often the first to notice any side effects caused by medication. In residential homes, care assistants will be aware of any changes of medication because they are usually responsible for giving out medication. In nursing homes, medication is given out by registered nurses. Care assistants, though, are often aware that medication has been changed. Care assistants who notice that an individual has become confused should inform a registered nurse in a nursing home, or the manager or a senior member of staff in a residential home.

Sometimes confusion creeps up slowly but staff should always check that there is no treatable physical cause before accepting confusion. Certain diseases such as diabetes, Parkinson's disease, thyroid disease and kidney disease can cause confusion. The registered nurse or doctor should be informed if an older person is becoming confused.

Mental illness and confusion

Many older people suffer from senile dementia. Dementia is not a disease but a label used to describe a cluster of symptoms. It is estimated that 25% of people over the age of 85 suffer from dementing illness. The commonest cause of dementia is Alzheimer's disease. This is a progressive mental illness. At first individuals become forgetful and muddled but eventually they become completely disorientated and unable to care for themselves. Individuals suffering from dementia are normally able to carry on living at home in the early stages of the disease. When the disease becomes more advanced they are admitted to residential and nursing homes. Normally individuals admitted to nursing homes are suffering from a more advanced stage of dementia than those in residential homes. Dementia is a progressive neurological disease that eventually leads to death.

Memory loss

Memory is lost in dementia. Short-term memory is most affected. The individual suffering from dementia may not be able to remember what he or she ate at lunchtime but can remember the events of long ago very clearly. It is important that the care assistant bears this in mind. An older person with Alzheimer's disease can often remember the names of close friends and family but forgets the care assistants' names. He or she may have to be shown the way back to the bedroom each time because short-term memory is so poor. People suffering from Alzheimer's disease can become very bewildered because they cannot remember where they are. The care assistant has an important role to play in gently reminding the older person of his or her whereabouts.

Wandering, shouting and screaming

Many older people with Alzheimer's disease appear to wander around without a purpose. They may shout out and scream. This is very distressing for care assistants and other patients. It is important to find out if there are reasons for the person's behaviour:

- Is the person in pain? Pain killers may help.
- Is the person constipated? Treatment will help.
- Is the individual hungry? Perhaps that walk to the kitchen is to get a snack.
- Is the person bored? Spending time doing something with the patient will help.
- Does the individual want to go for a walk? Imagine how you would feel after a few weeks sitting around in the home if you were used to being active.

Making sense of an individual's behaviour

Often confused people will do things that upset other residents, but if we take time to find out the reasons for the behaviour, we can improve the situation. An elderly confused lady was upsetting all the other patients because she was constantly taking their handbags and hiding them in her locker. She had no family or visitors. The care assistant looking after her brought in a handbag from home and put a comb, some lipstick, tissues and a few biscuits in the bag. The lady stopped taking other people's bags because she had one of her own.

Care assistants can, by taking time to talk to and listen to the older person, help them enjoy a good quality of life within the home. Care assistants should communicate their findings to more senior staff within homes so that these can be recorded and all staff are aware of information which improves care.

Golden rules for communicating with confused people

People with Alzheimer's and other forms of dementia have major difficulties communicating. You need to use all your skills to enable you to communicate. Communicating with people with dementia is hard work and cannot be rushed. If you do not have enough time to spend, then wait until later.

- Eliminate any distractions. Find a quiet place.
- Take time to communicate. Sit down and relax. If you appear hurried or harassed, the individual may become tense.
- Speak slowly and clearly.
- Only use one idea in each sentence.
- Use plain language and check that the person has understood. If not repeat the information in a slightly different way.
- Use short sentences.
- Do not give too many choices in one sentence. For example ask 'Would you like a bath?' not 'Would you like a bath or would you prefer to wash?'.
- Ask the person's family what methods of communication they have found most effective.

If you suspect that there are other barriers to communication, such as deafness or poor eyesight, inform a registered nurse within the nursing home, or your manager or a senior member of staff in the residential home. Then the individual can be helped, perhaps by having a hearing aid or new glasses.

Communicating with people who do not speak English

Some older people have come to the UK from abroad and have never learnt to speak English. Many other older people have learnt to speak English but because of a neurological condition such as a stroke or dementia have lost the ability to communicate in English. Many people understand more of a language than they can speak. The older person's family can help you to discover how much the person understands. Care assistants can rule a piece of paper into two columns and write words in English on one side; the older person's family and friends can write these words in the person's own language in the other column and this can be used to help communicate. A scrapbook full of pictures with the words written in English and the person's own language can help. Using a picture board, such as those used by stroke patients, can also help with communication.

Beware of using gestures. Before you use gestures check with the person's family that the gestures you use have the same meaning in that person's culture. If gestures are the same then use them. If gestures differ slightly, make a note of this. When it is important that staff and patient communicate accurately, perhaps when the person is feeling unwell or is attending an outpatient's appointment, ask if a member of the family can act as an interpreter. Finally, don't forget that facial expressions and touch are very important aids to understanding. Face the person so that you can be seen clearly and use touch to reinforce your words. It is important to sit down if the individual is seated. Getting down to the same level makes communication friendlier, less threatening and easier.

Living without language

We develop the ability to speak as babies. We learn by hearing our voices and those of our families. Some people who are born deaf do not learn to speak. Most people you will meet in nursing and residential homes will have lost their speech because of illness. Some people lose the ability to speak, known as aphasia. Loss of speech can occur suddenly when a person has a stroke, or slowly as dementia progresses. Some people who are no longer able to speak can use aids to enable them to communicate; others are no longer able to use aids. It is very important that you discover as much as possible about the person's remaining abilities. This enables you to work out ways of communicating.

Speech and language therapists

Speech and language therapists specialise in enabling people with communication problems to communicate. If you are caring for a person with communication problems who has not been assessed by a speech and language therapist suggest that a therapist is called. If you are managing a residential home, you can refer the person yourself. Speech and language therapists have an open referral system. This means that anyone, including the person with the problem, a relative or a care assistant, can request a visit.

The speech and language therapist visits and carries out an assessment of the person's abilities. If the person is frail, nervous or has profound problems communicating, the therapist may visit several times to complete the assessment. When the assessment is completed, the therapist will have worked out the person's problems and developed ways to enable communication to take place. The therapist will provide staff with information and suggestions based on the person's ability to communicate.

Aids to communication

Some people although unable to speak understand speech well. Cards with a single word or a commonly used phrase can help in such circumstances. Computers have the potential to revolutionise the lives of people with an intact intellect who lose the ability to speak. The person can type using fingers. If the person is unable to use their hands, even a pencil between the teeth enables the person to type words. In the US, scientists are developing systems that allow the person to blow a certain number of times for each letter. Research is being carried out on the use of eye movements to communicate. In the future, we will see computers used more to enable people to communicate.

Some people who are unable to speak also have difficulty reading. If the problem is poor vision, this is often easily corrected by using glasses. Sometimes cataracts clouding the vision are the problem. Cataracts can now be easily treated on a day surgery basis. Sometimes though, the problem is that the person can no longer make sense of written words. In such cases pictures can be used. In the past staff used to look through catalogues and magazines and pick out pictures. These were glued onto cards and used to help people communicate. Often the pictures were too small or difficult to obtain. Now computers can be used to prepare communication aids. Most homes now have computers and a third of the UK population has a computer at their own home. Clip art packages, once an expensive luxury, are now available for around £20. These can be used to produce large clear pictures. The pictures can be printed on to card and given to residents who have communication problems. If you do not have access to a computer at home or at work one of your colleagues or a relative may be able to help.

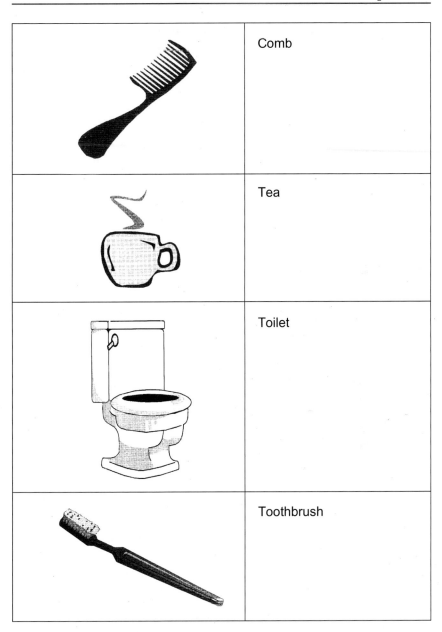

	Comb
	Tea
	Toilet
	Toothbrush

Fig. 2.1   Example of a communication card.

Using non verbal communication

Assessment gives you the information you need to develop ways to communicate. If the person is unable to read there is no point in writing things down. If the person is unable to see there is no point in providing pictures. If the person is unable to hear there is no point in speaking. The challenge then is to develop ways to enable you to communicate and to enable the person to communicate with you.

The speech and language therapist will be able to advise you of ways to communicate. Often touch is an important way of communicating and of reinforcing our words. Touch is very powerful. One research project a few years ago demonstrates this. The researcher left money on top of a telephone box and watched someone enter the booth. When the person came out the student asked if they had found her money. She touched half of the people on the arm as she asked her question. People who were touched were much more likely to return the money than those who were not. Touching someone gently on the arm is one way of breaking through the communication barriers that exist.

Developing relationships

The ability to communicate is so important to the development of relationships. Communication enables you to find out who the person is and how the person reacts. Relatives and friends can help you find out about the person who has communication problems. Often if these problems are long-standing, relatives and friends have developed ways to communicate. Develop relationships with the relatives and friends of those you care for and work with them to improve communication skills.

Maintaining relationships

Sometimes a person you are caring for loses the ability to communicate because of an illness such as stroke. The person may be able to understand everything you say but because she is unable to reply you no longer make the effort to communicate. This can be soul destroying. Don't assume that lack of response means lack of understanding. Continue to communicate and observe how the person responds. You may have to use some of the tips outlined earlier in the chapter to enable you to maintain communication.

Portfolio preparation

Your assessor will use a variety of methods to assess how effectively you communicate. The most popular methods of assessing a student's communication skills are direct observation and questioning. Your assessor may wish you to prepare written work when it is not possible to assess your skills in the workplace. Direct observation of communicating with a person who is unable to speak may not be possible because all the people in the home are able to speak. Written work can be used to assess your understanding of communication or to supplement the evidence gained by direct observation and questioning. Discuss portfolio preparation with your assessor before beginning any written work. Some suggestions for portfolio work are:

- Explain the ways we communicate. What difficulties do you face when communicating? How do you overcome these problems?
- Write a short case history about a person you have cared for. This should be 1–2 sides of A4 paper. Outline the communication difficulties and how these were overcome.
- Write one page of A4 paper about the importance of communication in care settings.

Further reading

These books may be available in your local or college library.

Counsel and Care (1993) *Sound Barriers* – a study of the needs of older people with hearing loss living in residential care and nursing homes. Available from the charity Counsel and Care, Twyman House, 16 Bonny Street, London NW1 9PG. Tel. 0171 485 1550.

Law, D. (1980) *Living After a Stroke*. Souvenir Press, London. This is a personal account of a woman's struggle to overcome the effects of her stroke.

Parr, S., Byng, S., Gilpin, S. & Ireland, C. (1998) *Talking about Aphasia*. Open University Press, Buckingham. This book is based on interviews with people who have had strokes. It explains what it is like to lose the ability to communicate.

Chapter 3

Health, Safety and Security

Introduction

This chapter covers the mandatory units CU1, CU1.1, CU1.2 and CU1.3 – 'promote monitor and maintain health, safety and security within the home'. Further details on moving and handling individuals can be found in Chapter 10. The aim of this chapter is to outline how you can contribute to maintaining the health and safety not only of older people but also of visitors and colleagues within the home.

This chapter includes information on:
- Safety and security within the home
- Who can enter the home
- The health and safety legislation – employer and employee responsibilities
- Action to be taken in the event of fire
- What to do if a resident is missing
- Preventing accidents
- Recording and learning lessons from accidents
- Identifying people at risk of accidents
- Balancing the risk of accident against the quality of life
- Restraint
- Medical emergencies

Safety and security within the home

Health and safety is now given more attention than before. Employers and managers are required to assess risks and act to reduce the risk of accidents occurring. Staff are required to comply with the health and safety policy in the home. Accidents are less likely to occur if every member of staff is aware of how accidents can occur and works to reduce the risk of accidents occurring. More details about this are given later in the chapter.

Older people living in homes and staff working within homes can be vulnerable to attack. There have been cases where intruders have entered homes and robbed and attacked staff and residents. In some cases, people have been seriously injured. In the past, many homes left the front entrance to the home 'on the latch' so that visitors could enter without having to be let in. Now the majority of homes have the front door closed and visitors must ring the doorbell. Some homes now use a combination lock. Visitors and staff are given the four digit combination and punch in the numbers to enter the home. These measures increase the safety and security of the people in the home. Staff are also more aware of who is in the building and this is important if a fire occurs. Some homes still leave a side entrance open during daylight hours. At night, it is the policy in most homes that doors are locked and ground floor windows (apart from fanlights) are closed. Check what policies your home has for ensuring security.

Who can enter the home

Nursing and residential homes are the homes of older people; they are not public places and there is no automatic right of entry for the public. In practice people who have a purpose in visiting the home, such as relatives and friends of patients and people who have come to deliver goods or services, are allowed free entry to the home. If a person living in the home does not wish to see someone (perhaps a neighbour), the neighbour has no right to enter the home.

Certain people have the legal right to enter the home:

- Registration officers
- Employees of the electricity board who may wish to read the meter
- Employees of the gas board who may wish to read the meter or investigate possible gas leaks
- Employees of the water board who may wish to read the water meter (most homes now have water meters and are charged according to how much water is used) or investigate possible water leaks
- Fire officers who are employed by the fire brigade and have the power to visit the home and check that fire precautions are satisfactory
- Members of the local fire brigade who may wish to familiarise themselves with the layout of the home – this enables them to evacuate patients quickly and safely if required because of a fire
- Health and safety officers employed to ensure that health and safety standards are met

- Environmental health officers who ensure that food handling and storage are satisfactory and that policies on waste disposal are satisfactory
- Pharmacists employed by the local NHS trust to ensure that medicines are stored and administered correctly

Although these groups of people have the legal right to enter the home, you should check the person's identification before allowing entry. There are reports of people claiming to be social workers or inspectors entering homes, assaulting residents and stealing their possessions.

Legal requirements

There are several laws governing health and safety in the workplace:

- Common law
- Health and Safety at Work Act 1974
- Management of Health & Safety at Work Regulations 1992, amended 1994
- Control of Substances Hazardous to Health 1988, known as COSHH
- Reporting of Injury, Disease and Dangerous Occurrences Regulations 1995, known as Riddor
- Manual Handling Operations Regulations 1992
- Fire Safety Regulations 1997

Common law

Common law has evolved over the last 1000 years and is unwritten. Under common law, each of us has a 'duty of care'. Employers, statutory bodies and professionals who breach this duty may be sued for negligence. The introduction of 'no win, no fee' cases means that people are now more likely to sue. In negligence claims the person suing must prove:

- That the company/person had a general duty of care to prevent foreseeable injuries
- That the failure to prevent injury was negligent
- That this failure caused the injury.

The case history below illustrates how negligence claims can work.

Case history

In 1996, a resident's bath oil was spilt on a vinyl 'non slip' floor. The care assistant bathing the resident accompanied the resident to her room. She did not mop up the bath oil, as she was busy; anyway, it was the last bath of the morning. Soon the domestic would come to clean the bathroom. Unfortunately, the domestic did not come soon enough. The resident's elderly visitor, noting that the bath oil had not been brought back from the bathroom went to fetch it. She slipped on the floor and fractured her femur. She sued the home for negligence. Her solicitor argued that the home was negligent in failing to prevent a foreseeable accident. The nursing home settled out of court on legal advice.

People whose actions have contributed to their injury may be found 'contributory negligent' and any damages awarded may be reduced.

Health and Safety at Work Act 1974

The Health and Safety at Work Act was introduced in 1974. The Act is the main piece of UK health and safety legislation and outlines broad principles concerning health and safety. Other more recent legislation is more specific. The key points of the Act are as follows.

The Act is a piece of criminal law. People who fail to comply with the Act can be prosecuted and fined or jailed if found guilty.

Employers' responsibilities

- Those who employ more than five people must prepare, review and revise a written health and safety policy. This should acknowledge and comply with legislation.
- Employers must ensure the health and safety of employees at work and other people on the premises.
- Employers must display a certificate of employer's liability insurance.
- Employers must display the poster *Health and Safety Law – what you should know* or distribute leaflets giving this information.
- Employers must ensure that employees receive adequate and appropriate information, instruction and training to carry out their work safely.

Employee responsibilities

- Employees must comply with legislation and ensure that their actions do not adversely affect others.

■ Employees are entitled to sue their employers if they have been injured in the course of their work.

Self employed people (such as the window cleaner) must comply with legislation and ensure that their actions do not adversely affect others.

Manufacturers and suppliers must ensure that their products are safe when used properly. They must provide health and safety information about their products.

Management of Health and Safety at Work Regulations

The Management of Health and Safety at Work Regulations 1992 were amended in 1994 by the Management of Health and Safety at Work (Amendment) Regulations. These regulations require employers to carry out risk assessments. The key points of the Regulations are as follows.

Employers are required to:

■ Assess risks associated with the business to determine how to eliminate or minimise those risks.

■ Take action to eliminate or minimise risk.

■ Appoint 'competent persons' to help meet the requirements. This can be the manager or a member of staff. If no one within the home has the skills then consultants can be used.

■ Ensure that temporary staff (including agency staff) are informed of any health and safety information and/or the skills necessary to do their job.

■ Consider the capabilities of each individual to do their work safely.

The aim of the legislation is to ensure that the employer takes care to ensure the health and safety of employees and people living in or entering the home, such as by taking precautions to reduce accidents. This means that if an employer is aware of some problem that may cause an accident, steps should be taken to prevent accidents occurring. If the employer knows that a carpet is frayed and could cause someone to trip but does not act, a breach of the Act has occurred. There have been cases where employers have been prosecuted for failing to clear snow from paths because accidents have occurred.

Employers who have more than five employees are required to have a policy statement. This details the employer's responsibilities and the staff's responsibilities. The policy statement may give details about special precautions to be taken to prevent accidents; for example, it may be policy for domestic staff to leave signs saying 'Caution wet floor' on floors that they have just mopped. The policy statement may also give detailed instructions about the safekeeping of items such as cleaning materials and medicines. It will also instruct all employees about action they should take if they become aware of a hazard or a breach of the health and safety policy.

Employers have a duty to provide equipment to prevent accidents. This means that employers should provide a range of equipment, from rubber gloves and overalls for domestics required to clean toilets, to hoists for staff required to move residents.

Employees are required to:

- Adhere to the instructions, policies and procedures laid down by their employer.
- Report any shortcomings in the employer's arrangements; for example, if there are instructions that Mrs X is to be moved using the hoist but the hoist is broken.

Staff working within the home have duties and responsibilities to work in ways that reduce the risk of accidents and make the home as safe as possible.

New and expectant mothers

The workplace can damage the health of mothers and of their unborn children. Research shows that working long hours, working shifts, heavy physical labour and stress can affect pregnancy. The 1994 amendment regulations recognise that new and expectant mothers are particularly vulnerable in the workplace. Employers must carry out specific risk assessment that includes the risks to expectant mothers, new mothers and mothers who are breast feeding. The Health and Safety Executive produces guidance. Staff must inform employers when they become pregnant, are breast feeding or have recently given birth. This enables the employer to meet legal requirements.

Documentation

The approach to record keeping which courts of law adopt tends to be 'if it is not recorded it has not been done'. Record keeping enables the home to demonstrate that staff have worked safely. Further information on record keeping is given in Chapter 5.

Training

Employers are required to provide adequate training of staff to prevent accidents. In homes, this will mean that staff who are required to move residents should have regular instruction and updating in moving and handling; further details are given in Chapter 10. The Care Standards Bill 2000 states that all staff must have health and safety training as part of their induction. Employers have a duty to ensure that staff are aware of what action they must take during emergencies of:

- Fire
- Accident
- A missing resident.

Cleaning materials

Many cleaning materials are very toxic. Bleach and toilet cleaners can damage the skin and cause serious injury if drunk. Other cleaning materials may not appear dangerous but can cause accidents; for example, spilt washing-up liquid can cause a fall. In residential homes, care assistants may be responsible for cleaning as well as caring. Staff should ensure that all cleaning materials are kept locked away. It may be convenient to have the toilet cleaner by the side of the toilet but this could cause serious harm to a confused patient.

Nursing homes normally employ domestic staff but you may find cleaning materials left out. You have a duty to remove these from patient areas to prevent the possibility of injury.

Medications

In nursing homes, medicines are stored in a locked cabinet and only registered nurses have access to the drugs cupboard or trolley. Medicines that are being returned to the pharmacy are often stored in the treatment room. Creams and lotions are also stored in the treatment room. Treatment rooms are locked. You should make sure you always lock treatment room doors after leaving. In some homes some residents keep their own medicines and take them when prescribed. If the older person leaves her medicine lying around there is a danger that a confused patient might take these medicines. If you are worried about such a situation, consult your manager.

Fire training

Every person working in the home should be aware of what to do in case of fire. Each person working in the home should be given training in this and should attend a fire drill every six months. It is important that you are aware of where each fire exit is and what to do in case of fire.

Normally when the fire alarm goes off all staff report to a fire assembly point. Find out where the fire assembly point is in your home. It is usually by the main panel of the fire alarm. The fire alarm in homes normally has one large panel and a number of smaller panels. The home is divided into zones and the rooms and areas covered by each zone will be written on the fire panel; for example, zone one might be the lounge, kitchen, and laundry. If a fire has occurred in zone one staff would check in which part of this area the fire had occurred. If the fire alarm has been triggered in the kitchen by burning toast the action taken would be different from that required if the deep fat fryer was in flames.

Find out if your home has written guidance on what action is to be taken in case of fire. Many homes have this guidance framed and hung on the wall next to fire alarm panels.

Fire exits

All fire exits in the home should be clearly marked and should be kept clear at all times. It is easy though for busy staff to allow fire exits to become blocked. A delivery of stationery or goods may be left blocking a fire exit as staff intend to put things away later. Relatives can easily place a chair in front of the fire exit in the lounge and then leave without putting it back. Homes are for living in but it is important that carers are aware that blocked exits cause delay in evacuating the home if a fire breaks out. At times, staff must exercise great tact in ensuring that residents and their families are not offended, but that exits are kept clear.

Accident policy

The aim of all accident policies is to prevent accidents occurring whenever possible. It is not possible to make any home completely safe and this will be discussed later in the chapter. You can contribute to safety within the home by reporting anything that is likely to cause an accident and by taking action, wherever possible, to prevent accidents occurring. This will be discussed later in the chapter.

Missing resident

The home should have a policy on action to be taken if a resident goes missing. If the person tends to go out unaccompanied, suggest that the individual carry identification in case of accident. A note tucked into a wallet or purse saying 'Mrs Doris Swan is a resident of Eastways Residential Home; in case of accident please telephone...' will help ensure that the home is contacted if an accident occurs.

If the person tends to wander and may have left the home in a confused state, the home should have a policy for dealing with this. Normally such a policy involves both calling the police and staff searching for the older person. It is possible for the individual to get some distance from the home very quickly. An older person dressed in ordinary clothes will not attract any attention. Many bus drivers do not ask to see bus passes when a person is obviously above retirement age. The police will find it difficult to locate a lady of 83 with white hair and glasses wearing a flowered Marks and Spencer's dress!

Many homes now take photographs of residents. A photograph is often attached to the medication chart to enable temporary staff to identify residents. In some homes, photographs of patients are put on their bedroom doors. This helps residents, visitors and staff to find a person's room. If the person goes missing and the police have a recent photograph, their job becomes much easier.

Accidents

Preventing accidents

You can contribute to safety within the home by reporting anything that is likely to cause an accident, and by acting wherever possible to prevent accidents occurring. Some factors that can cause or contribute to accidents are given here.

Environmental hazards

A wet floor can be slippery and can cause a fall. A toilet that is dark because the light bulb does not work and has not been replaced can make it difficult for the older person to see where she is going and can cause a fall. A building that is poorly maintained can lead to accidents.

Equipment that is not working properly can also cause accidents. If you discover that the brakes on a patient's wheelchair are not working, remove the wheelchair and report the problem so that repairs can be organised quickly. Homes should have a spare wheelchair that can be used to transport residents who are ill, or can be used temporarily by a patient whose wheelchair is unsafe.

Objects left carelessly on the floor may not be noticed by older people, who can fall over. Remove any hazards, wherever possible, and inform the person in charge of the home at once. Inadequate seating can lead to some disabled people falling out of chairs. Some older people living in nursing homes are very disabled and are unable to sit in ordinary armchairs. It is now possible to buy chairs specially designed to enable these people to sit comfortably in chairs that will support them. An example of one of these is given in Fig. 3.1a. Specially designed chairs provide support for disabled older people but do not restrain or restrict the person in any way (Fig. 3.1b).

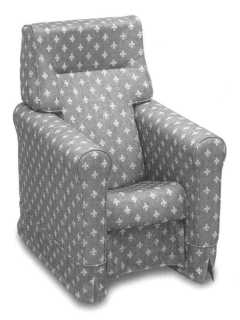

Fig. 3.1(a)   Example of a specially designed chair to enable a disabled person to sit comfortably.

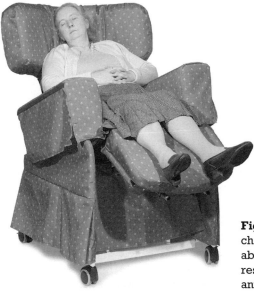

Fig. 3.1(b)   Specially designed chairs provide support for disabled older people but do not restrain or restrict the person in any way.

Unsuitable footwear

Unsuitable footwear can make it difficult to walk and can lead to accidents. Many older people, especially those who have not been walking around, find that their feet swell. This can make it difficult to find shoes that fit properly. Some older people have deformed feet; bunions and arthritis can cause foot deformities. These deformities can make it very difficult for older people to find shoes that fit properly. Special shoes can be made for patients who have difficulty in wearing ordinary shoes. The patient's GP writes to the surgical fitter (known as an orthotist) and asks for shoes to be made for the person. The orthotist visits, measures the person's feet, and discusses which type and colour of shoes or boots the person would prefer. These are made specially and the orthotist returns to fit them when they are ready.

Some older people, particularly those who have suffered from strokes, require a calliper to provide support. These are supplied by the orthotist. Sometimes special shoes are made and the calliper is designed to fit into the heel of the shoe. Sometimes the older person's own shoes are adapted so that the calliper will fit.

People who suffer from arthritis of the knee may find that one of their knees tends to 'give'. A knee support, supplied by the orthotist, can prevent this. People who have broken a leg may have one leg shorter than the other because of surgery. Special shoes can be made to correct this and enable the older person to walk normally.

If the older person has been supplied with special footwear or an aid such as a calliper, you may need to help them put it on. Older people who have suitable footwear are less likely to have accidents.

Clothing

Clothing can cause accidents. Many older women prefer full length nightdresses and dressing gowns. If these are too long, the individual can trip over and fall. Many male patients wear pyjamas and can easily fall if the legs are too long.

How accidents affect older people

Accidents can have serious consequences. The older person can lose confidence because of a fall and this can cause them to walk less and to become weaker. Sometimes the older person who falls fractures a bone; if she puts out a hand to save herself the wrist may fracture, known as a Colles' fracture. The thigh bones (femurs) or the top of the thigh bone (shaft of femur) can also become fractured as a result of a fall.

Older people often suffer from a condition known as

osteoporosis, which causes the bones to become thinner, weaker and more easily broken. Figs. 3.2 and 3.3 show healthy bone and bone where osteoporosis has weakened the bone.

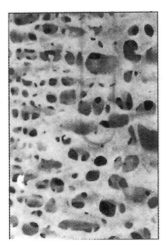

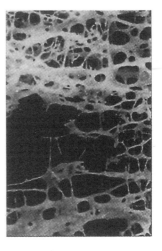

Fig. 3.2 Healthy bone.

Fig. 3.3 Bone weakened by osteoporosis.

Discovering who is at risk of having accidents

People living in homes have a wide range of abilities. Some have few problems in walking whilst others require aids and help to move around. Some residents are alert whilst others are not. Some individuals see well whilst others have very poor vision. Some of the people living in your home will be much more likely to have accidents than others.

Homes aim to enable older people to live their lives as they would wish if they were at home. The aim of care within homes should be to reduce the risk of accidents and to protect individuals who are at risk of having accidents. Most homes now assess residents to discover who is most at risk of having an accident. If the person is at risk this is noted in the care plan along with action to be taken to reduce risks. It is important to realise that no home can be made totally safe and that no one can guarantee that accidents will not happen.

Balancing risks and quality of life

Living is about taking risks. We all take risks every day of our lives. We risk crossing the road where there are no traffic lights; we take risks every time we step into a car or on a bus, or take part in sports. Yet if we stayed at home and took no risks life would not be worth living. When we take risks we weigh up the risk and decide on the possible gains and losses from taking that risk.

In homes staff must balance the duty of care and the possibility of trying so hard to avoid accidents that we risk making the older person's life a misery by preventing her from living life to the full. The care assistant who left a confused resident alone and unsupervised in the bath knowing that she was not capable of calling for help would be failing in her duty of care. Another individual recovering from illness might ask you to sit with her while she bathes because she is feeling nervous. Another individual might wish to bath in private and may ask you to leave after she has been helped into the bath.

It is important to treat people as individuals; older people are just like us, only older. Some older people who are recovering from illness are determined to 'get back on their feet'. In the process of regaining mobility and strength, the person may fall many times. Staff should respect the individual's wishes and offer support, help and encouragement.

Restraint

It is illegal to restrain anyone without their consent. It is also illegal to restrain any person on another person's instructions. In some homes, you may see different types of restraint used, including bed rails, tables and lockers.

Bed rails
Bed rails were used routinely in hospitals until a few years ago. Some hospitals had policies that stated that all individuals over a certain age were to have bed rails fitted to their beds to prevent falls. We now know that bed rails can lead to serious injury and they are only used in special circumstances.

Bed rails prevent individuals getting up and this can lead to incontinence. When bed rails are used some older people become depressed and upset, and this can affect their mental and physical health and lead to them becoming weaker and sicker. Some people climb over bed rails and can fall. There have been reports of people who caught an arm or leg in the bed rail, struggled to get free and broke a limb. The bed rail, which is designed to prevent accidents, can actually cause them.

Tables, chairs and lockers
These can be used to barricade the person into bed making it

difficult or impossible for them to get out, but using furniture in this way can lead to accidents.

Preventing the older person falling out of bed

Staff often worry that if a person falls the staff will be blamed and everyone will think the person has been neglected. Homes that have risk assessment policies will have these documented and patients, staff, relatives and registration officers will be aware of these policies. Older people do not normally fall out of bed and many staff worry unnecessarily about them doing so. You can reduce the risk of accidents at night by:

- Making sure that the patient can reach the call bell
- Assuring the person that staff are there to help and that they should not hesitate to ring if help is required
- Answering bells promptly
- Making sure the person does not feel rushed or a 'nuisance'
- Leaving a light on so that if the person wishes to get up in the night, she can see
- Leaving the room tidy and not leaving any obstacles which could cause a fall
- Leaving any aids such as a walking frame and shoes where the person can reach them.

Recording accidents

All accidents that occur in the home must be recorded in an accident book. The type of record kept varies from area to area. There are no national guidelines stating how these records should be kept. In practice accident records that satisfy the local inspection team are kept. In some areas, a form is issued in triplicate; one form is kept in the patient's notes, another in an accident folder and another is placed in the care plan. In other areas, all accidents are recorded in a bound book. Find out the policy for recording accidents in your home.

Learning from accidents

Some accidents that occur could, with hindsight, have been prevented. In other cases, perhaps involving faulty equipment or poor handling techniques, accidents may recur if action is not taken. In some homes senior staff discuss and review accidents so that, wherever possible, lessons can be learnt and further accidents prevented.

Medical emergencies

All staff working in care homes come face to face with emergencies from time to time. It is important that you have some basic knowledge of first aid. The aims of first aid are to:

- Preserve life
- Prevent the emergency worsening
- Help recovery

What to do if you find a patient has collapsed

- First take a deep breath and remain calm
- Use the call bell to call for help
- Check what is happening – is the patient conscious or unconscious? How serious is the situation?

The most important things you can do can be remembered by 'ABC'. Ensure that the person's:

- **A**irway is open and he is able to breathe
- **B**reathing is taking place
- **C**irculation is satisfactory

Airway obstruction

The airway enables us to breathe air in and out of our lungs. It can become obstructed for a number of reasons, but the commonest causes of airway obstruction are choking or loss of consciousness.

If the person is choking this could be because food or dentures are blocking the airway. The person may have vomited and vomit has collected at the back of the throat. Open the person's mouth gently. Use two fingers to feel around for any food, vomit, or dentures that may be causing the person to choke. Remove anything that is blocking the airway.

If the person is unable to speak and is turning blue use the Heimlichs manoeuvre which is shown in Fig. 3.4.

There are many reasons for loss of consciousness, including strokes, fits and diabetes. Staff who know as much about the older person's condition as possible can respond more effectively. People who become unconscious should be placed in the recovery position (Fig. 3.5). You may require help to place a person in this position. If possible remove the person's dentures as they may slip in the mouth and block the airway. Loosen tight clothing and call for help immediately.

Breathing

Some older people suffer from asthma and carry inhalers that help them to breathe more easily. It is important that you find out

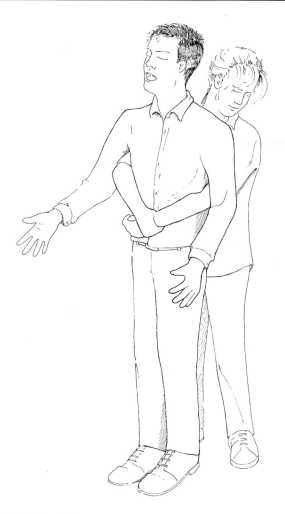

Fig. 3.4 Heimlich manoeuvre.

whether any of the people in the home where you work suffer from asthma. If a person in the home does suffer from asthma and may require help to use an inhaler if he or she has become breathless, find out how to do this before an emergency occurs. If the person is having difficulty breathing but is conscious, help him to sit up. Loosen any tight clothing, such as a tie, shirt collar or belt. People who have difficulty breathing feel very frightened and this fear makes breathing more difficult. Do your best to reassure the person as this will help prevent breathing problems worsening. Ask the person to take slow deep breaths, and seek assistance.

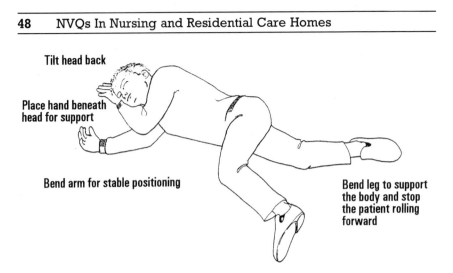

Tilt head back

Place hand beneath head for support

Bend arm for stable positioning

Bend leg to support the body and stop the patient rolling forward

Fig. 3.5   Recovery position.

Circulation

If a person becomes unconscious, it is important to be able to decide quickly if the situation is a life threatening emergency or simply a faint:

■ Check the person's colour – blue or grey skin indicates a life threatening emergency
■ Check breathing – is the person breathing at all, with difficulty or normally
■ Check the pulse – is the pulse absent or does it appear weak

If the person's skin colour is abnormal or breathing is absent, or the person is breathing with difficulty, or the pulse is absent or weak, call for help immediately. This is a medical emergency perhaps caused by a stroke or heart attack. Check that the airway is clear and place the person in the recovery position while waiting for help.

Fainting is a brief loss of consciousness. People who have fainted may appear very pale but their skin does not become blue or grey. Breathing is normal and the pulse is always present, though it can appear weak. Fainting can occur in adults of all ages. It may be caused by hunger, shock or even getting up too quickly. The person faints because the brain is not receiving sufficient blood. A person who has fainted should not be sat up because sitting up reduces the flow of blood to the brain.

If you find a person unconscious, it is important to check their colour. Clothing should be loosened and the person should lie down until she feels well enough to sit up. Drinking from a glass of cold water may help the person to feel better.

Chest pain

Chest pain and circulation problems can be caused by angina or a heart attack. In both cases, the heart muscle will not be getting sufficient blood and oxygen. If the person is unconscious, place them in the recovery position. If the individual is conscious, help her to breathe by sitting her up and loosening clothing. Call for help at once.

If the person is known to have a heart condition, their GP may have prescribed tablets or a spray of the drug glycerine trinitrate. This drug acts by helping the arteries that bring blood to the heart to expand, which improves the supply of blood to the heart.

Check if any of the patients in the home where you work are known to have a heart condition. If anyone has been prescribed glycerine trinitrate by a GP find out how this is given in an emergency before the emergency occurs.

Bleeding

Bleeding can be caused by a fall. If the patient is bleeding, remain calm. A clean towel or item of clothing can be applied to the wound and pressure applied to control bleeding. A sterile dressing pack can be fetched when help arrives, and the wound can be cleaned and examined to decide what further treatment is required.

Suspected fractures

The aim of first aid is to prevent movement of the injured part of the body and to arrange for the person to be transferred to hospital as soon as possible. In some cases, it is obvious that a person has fractured and patients with obvious fractures are sent to hospital at once by ambulance. Before your manager dials 999 for an ambulance, you need to know:

- What happened?
- Where is the pain?

The ambulance staff answering the emergency call will require this information.

If you have any suspicion that the person has fractured, do not move them. Ambulance paramedics will support the limb before moving the person.

- Do not give the person anything to eat or drink, as emergency surgery may be required
- It is important to keep the person warm   place a blanket over them

■ If the person is bleeding, apply direct pressure to the wound to control bleeding

Burns and scalds

Burns are caused by dry heat; scalds are caused by hot liquids. The treatment of burns and scalds is the same. The aims of first aid in this case are to:

■ Stop the pain
■ Relieve pain and swelling
■ Prevent infection

You should:

■ Assess the severity of the burn and call for professional help
■ Place the burnt area under cold running water for at least ten minutes
■ If the hand has been burnt remove rings and watches if possible
■ Do not try to remove clothing which may be stuck to the skin
■ Do not apply any creams to the burn
■ Do not burst blisters
■ Do not apply a dressing to the burn – this may stick and cause further damage
■ If the burn is severe the skin can be wrapped in cling film or placed in a clean plastic bag until help arrives

Learning more about first aid

All care assistants should have some basic knowledge of first aid. Sometimes it is possible to take a first aid course as part of your NVQ training. If you are working in a residential home in a senior capacity, you will require training to equip you with the skills needed to cope in an emergency. Care assistants working in nursing homes may also benefit from such training. The St John Ambulance run first aid courses locally and further details can be obtained from:

Medical Department
St John Ambulance
1 Grosvenor Crescent
London SW1X 7EF
Tel. 020 7235 5231

Summary

Staff working in homes should aim to provide an environment that is as safe as possible for older people. There is, however, no such thing as a 'safe' environment. Staff should work with older people and support them in living their lives as they wish. Many homes have policies that help determine the risk of people falling or having accidents. Accidents should be recorded and where possible action should be taken to prevent similar accidents occurring.

Portfolio preparation _____

Your assessor must have evidence that you can meet the performance criteria for this unit. Before beginning this unit discuss assessment strategies with your assessor. Most of the evidence for this unit can be gained by direct observation of your work. You may be asked to provide the following types of evidence:

- Products. This might be a copy of a hazard report you completed after identifying a hazard. It could be a note in a resident's notes giving details of how you dealt with an accident. It could be details of a first aid dressing that you have applied to a colleague after an accident.
- Witness testimony. This is a statement from a senior member of staff. It might be a statement detailing how you have met certain performance criteria.
- Written work. You might be asked to prepare a piece of work about the factors that increase the risk of accidents occurring.

Your assessor may also use other methods to help you gain evidence for this unit. These may include:

- Verbal questioning
- Written questions
- Simulations to demonstrate that you have the skills to work effectively in emergencies.

Further information

Health & Safety at Work Act 1974, The Stationery Office, London. Your home will probably have a copy of the Act; if not, the local reference library or your college library will have one.

Health and Safety Executive (1974) *A Guide to the Health and Safety at Work Act 1974*. HSE Books, Sheffield.
Tel. 0541 545 5000
The Health and Safety Executive produces a range of leaflets on health and safety. These include guidance on risk assessment and legal requirements. Copies can be obtained by writing to:
HSE Information Centre
Broad Lane
Sheffield S3 7HQ
The HSE have a website and all their publications can be down-loaded from this site:
http://www.open.gov.uk/hse/hsehome.htm

Fire safety. The local fire station will have a number of videos that you may find of interest. Fire brigade staff use these when giving talks to various groups. One video that you may find interesting is *Hospitals Do Not Just Burn Down*. This video was made about 16 years ago but is still useful. The fire station may lend you this video but will require identification before doing so.

CTV
Low Burnham Hall
Halgarth
Nr Epworth
Doncaster DN9 1DE
Tel. 01427 874294
CTV have released a training video aimed at staff working in nursing and residential homes. Your home or college may have one that you can borrow.

Further reading

Counsel & Care (1993) *The Right to Take Risks*. Counsel & Care, London.
St John Ambulance, British Red Cross Society and St Andrew's Ambulance Association (1997) *First Aid Manual*, 7th edn. Dorling Kindersley, London.

Chapter 4

Protecting Individuals from Abuse

Introduction

This chapter covers the core units Z1, Z1.1, Z1.2 and Z1.3 – 'contribute to the protection of individuals from abuse'. This unit is common to all NVQ level 2 and level 3 units because abuse can occur in all care settings. This unit, because of its breadth, causes assessors and students great problems. Like all other units, you are required to demonstrate competence in all the elements of the units. Some assessors think that if the student does not actually witness abuse then they cannot complete the unit. They are mistaken. Students must demonstrate that they have the skills and knowledge to deal with abuse if it occurs. Students must demonstrate an awareness of the reasons why abuse occurs and work to provide a healthy work environment. Abuse is unacceptable and if detected must be dealt with. Abuse is shameful; it is not an educational opportunity.

Abuse of older people was first recognised 25 years ago but even today some homes do not have specific policies that prevent abuse from occurring or outline action to be taken in the event of abuse.

This chapter gives information on:

- The different types of abuse including:
  - Physical abuse
  - Passive abuse
  - Abuse of medications
  - Psychological abuse
  - Financial abuse
  - Sexual abuse
- Factors that increase the likelihood of abuse
- How to identify the residents most at risk of abuse
- Warning signs of abuse
- Action to take if abuse is occurring in your home
- Legal rights of older people living in homes caring for confused residents
- Caring for residents who wander
- Coping with older people who shout and scream
- Caring for people who are aggressive

What is abuse?

There are many definitions of abuse. The most commonly used are:

'A single or repeated act occurring within a relationship where there is an expectation of trust, which causes harm to an individual over the age of 65.'
'Abuse may range from a spontaneous act of frustration to the systematic terrorising of an older person.'

Elder abuse is mistreatment of an older person. It can, as the definitions show, be a single act or a long-term pattern of abuse. Abuse can have a long-term effect on the older person's physical and mental health. Many people when they hear the term abuse immediately think of physical abuse. There are a number of other types of abuse as well.

Physical abuse

Physical abuse ranges from deliberately hitting and hurting the older person through to neglect. The person abused may be hit or slapped. She may be handled roughly and may develop bruises on forearms and shins as a result. She may be pulled or pushed.

Passive abuse

Passive abuse is the term used when the older person's needs are neglected. Their needs may be unmet: the call bell may be 'dropped' on the floor out of the person's reach; the walking frame may be too far away for the person to reach it. These acts effectively cut the person off and prevent her from moving around or calling for help.

Aids that the older person depends on may be 'lost' or the person may not be able to reach them without help: without a hearing aid, the person cannot hear; without glasses, she may be unable to see; and without teeth, she will have great difficulty eating. The individual may not be helped to wash or bathe. In some cases people are left in night-clothes during the day or dressed in shabby, soiled clothing. The person who requires help to eat or drink may not receive it and may become dehydrated and ill as a result. Neglect affects a person emotionally and physically.

In many cases passive abuse occurs because staff have not received sufficient training and have not developed the skills required to help care for the older person. In other cases, staff do not receive sufficient supervision and support. But even in the best of environments, where staff are well educated and supported, abuse can occur. That is why it is so important that homes have procedures to detect abuse quickly.

Abuse of medications

Abuse of medications may occur when staff are unable to meet the person's needs and ask medical staff to prescribe sedatives. The older person who is wandering around the home upsetting other residents has a reason for wandering. Educated staff who are aware of this will try to find out the reason. The older person may be hungry, cold, searching for a book or a handbag, or may simply be bored. Giving a sedative solves nothing. The person will continue to walk around because his needs remain unmet. Now, however, because he has been sedated he is at greater risk of falling and injuring himself.

Professionals are increasingly aware that prescribing sedatives in an attempt to control behaviour can lead to many problems. Sedatives are prescribed less often than before. Staff need to observe people who are prescribed sedatives carefully. Sedatives can build up in the body gradually and the person can become too drowsy to eat, drink or function normally. If you notice such symptoms report them immediately.

Psychological abuse

Psychological abuse is shouting, swearing, laughing at, humiliating, ignoring, or frightening an older person. The abused person can be bullied, isolated and denied basic rights such as the right to privacy and dignity. Psychological abuse can affect the older person to just as great an extent as physical abuse. Carers should be sensitive to the older person's feelings, as a thoughtless comment can cause great offence to an older person living in the home.

Financial abuse

Financial abuse is stealing an older person's money or belongings. The abuse may be carried out by a member of staff, a member of the family or a 'friend'. The older person may be duped into signing papers giving access to savings or property. She may be asked to give valuable jewellery to a carer, relative or 'friend' for safekeeping.

Older people who have their nursing home fees met by either the Department of Social Security (DSS) or the local council receive a 'personal allowance'. Before the introduction of the Community Care Act, some residents agreed to spend part of this allowance on paying the home's fees if they were above DSS levels. When the Community Care Act was introduced in April 1993 Social Services Departments (SSDs) became responsible for paying for the care of people who had less than £16,000 in savings. In most parts of the country SSDs made it clear, when entering into contracts with homes, that they would meet the home's fees and that the individual was to have their personal allowance to spend as they wished. The Department of Health has now issued guidance supporting this. Under both DSS and SSD payment systems, the personal allowance is usually paid on a pension book. Many older people living in homes are unable to cash this personally at the local post office and rely on a relative to do this. In some circumstances, a senior member of staff at the home may do it. In some circumstances either relatives or staff members may defraud the older person of this money. Financial abuse includes theft of an older person's money, valuables or possessions. Good record keeping protects staff from allegations of financial abuse and enables homes to detect theft if it occurs. This is covered in detail in Chapter 5 on record keeping.

Sexual abuse

Sexual abuse is forcing an older person to take part in any sexual activity without consent. Sexual abuse occurs when an older person is involved in sexual activities to which they have not consented or, if they are in a confused state, do not truly comprehend. Sexual abuse includes inappropriate touching, fondling, kissing, oral contact, genital contact, digital penetration, rape, and being forced to watch videos or read pornographic magazines. Residents can be sexually abused by staff, relatives or visitors.

Who is most at risk of abuse?

Abuse in caring situations has been recognised for some time. Abuse is rare in settings where people are alert. It occurs more frequently when staff are caring for people who are unable to protect themselves or to protest. The typical victim is:

- Female
- Over 80 years old
- Physically dependent on staff
- Requiring high levels of care
- May have communication problems
- May be confused

Not all older people who are abused fit into the categories given above. Any older person is at risk of abuse. Research has shown that older people living in homes who require high levels of care are particularly at risk. Older people who are 'difficult' and whom staff find it a strain to care for are at risk. People who have communication problems are at greater risk of abuse than those who are able to communicate and build relationships with staff. People with communication problems are more vulnerable to abuse because they are usually unable to report the abuse.

Who abuses older people?

The literature on abuse states that the typical abuser is female, middle-aged and usually the offspring of the abused.

It is important not to be blinded by stereotypes. The person who abuses the older person is usually someone the older person knows well, a person who in normal circumstances the older person could trust. Relatives may abuse the person during visits. This abuse can be physical or psychological. In some cases relatives can bring medication from home and give this to the older person. Sometimes relatives can persuade or intimidate the older person into signing over property or valuables or into giving away jewellery. 'Friends' may abuse the older person. A member of staff may abuse the older person and could be anyone who comes into contact with them: a domestic, a carer or a registered nurse.

Possible signs that abuse is occurring

In the last few years there have been reports of abuse occurring in hospitals and nursing and residential homes. Although abuse is rare, one case is too many. It is important to be aware of the signs of abuse, as given below.

Signs of physical abuse

- Unexplained injuries: bruising, particularly to shins and forearms, cuts and tears to skin, burns
- Signs of overmedication
- Signs of the person not having prescribed medication
- The person is quiet and withdrawn
- The person is nervous and eager to please
- Poor hygiene – the person may be dirty and smelly
- Poor diet – the person may be very undernourished and thin
- Insufficient fluids – the person may be very dehydrated

- Isolation – the person may be left in her room and may be unable to move out of it without help
- The person is unable to call for help as she has no access to a call bell
- Aids are 'forgotten' or lost

Indicators of sexual abuse

Sexual abuse is so dreadful that most of us would rather not think about it. It is important to be aware of the indicators of abuse so that if abuse occurs it can be detected and stopped. The indicators of sexual abuse are:

- Bleeding from the vagina or rectum
- Frequent vaginal infections
- Sexually transmitted diseases
- Bruising on the inner thighs
- Swelling and bruising in the genital area
- Sudden onset of confusion
- Nightmares
- Terror
- Depression
- Frequently talking about sex
- Discharge on underwear

Why abuse can occur in homes

Abuse within homes is completely unacceptable. It is more likely to occur in poorly managed homes; in homes where there are insufficient staff to meet older people's needs staff are under greater pressure. In some homes, staff are expected to give care they have not been trained to give and may find themselves 'out of their depth'. In other homes, staff may feel that they cannot turn to registered nurses or their manager for help and advice. In some homes, carers do not receive sufficient supervision.

Older people now living in nursing and residential homes are more acutely ill than before and require greater amounts of care. In some homes training and education programmes (such as NVQ courses) have been introduced. Abuse is more likely to occur in homes where staff feel overworked, unsupported and unable to cope and receive little training and education. It is important though to be aware that abuse can happen in even the best run homes. The home may, despite checks, inadvertently employ someone with a history of abuse to care for residents. The home may admit a resident who has been abused at home by a relative or 'friend'; if staff are not alert abuse may continue unchecked in the home.

What to do if abuse occurs

In some situations, the inexperienced care assistant may be unsure if an older person is being abused. You may witness a colleague appearing to argue with an older person but it may be that the colleague and the older person are teasing each other. In another situation, you may feel that a colleague is refusing to help an older person, for example:

'Mary get a wheelchair and wheel me downstairs please...'
'Why don't you get your walking stick and I'll walk down with you Mr Blackburn.'

In this case the care assistant may be encouraging Mr Blackburn to maintain his independence and to continue walking. If you feel unsure in such situations, you could ask the person who is with you. Many care assistants who are new to the home do not wish to risk upsetting staff. Find someone in the home you can trust, perhaps the matron or manager and ask, 'Does Mr Blackburn normally walk to the lounge?' You may discover that Mr Blackburn has come to the home for a period of convalescence, has lost confidence in his ability to walk, and needs support and encouragement.

In other cases, sadly, there can be no doubt that a colleague's behaviour is unacceptable and the older person is being abused. You may be on a placement or may be a new member of staff. You may fear that you will be seen as a trouble maker and that you will suffer as a result of reporting the abuse. You cannot ignore it; you must tell someone. The older person may be unable to tell staff what is happening; they may be too frightened to speak out. If you turn a blind eye the abuse will continue and may get worse.

Most homes take the issue of abuse very seriously. Most homes have a policy on action to take if abuse is suspected. This should be in the home's procedure book. This will give you information and advice about what to do if you suspect abuse. Normally you should ask to speak to the matron or manager and discuss the situation. Action can then be taken. If you do not feel able to approach the manager perhaps you could send a letter or leave a note giving information about the situation. Even if you are not able to sign the note, at least you will have informed the manager. If no action is taken or if you do not feel able to approach the manager, you can contact the registration and inspection unit for the home.

Nursing homes are inspected by the local health authority. If you ring the local hospital, they will give you the number of the registration unit. Residential homes are inspected by the registration and inspection unit run by social services. If you ring the local town hall, they will give you the number of the unit. From

2002 all homes will be inspected by the Commission for Care Standards. You can inform the registration unit of your concerns; your call will be in complete confidence and the inspection unit will investigate. Even if you do not wish to leave your name, the call will still be treated seriously.

You can, if you prefer, inform the person's care manager of the situation. Details of who the older person's care manager is should be recorded in the person's records. You may wish to call a helpline for advice and support. Details of these are given at the end of the chapter.

Abuse – the legal position

It is unlawful to abuse a person. Criminal charges can be brought against the abuser under the Offences Against the Person Act 1861. There are plans to update this law and the Law Commission recently issued a report recommending changes. If a registered nurse is accused of abuse the governing body for nursing staff, the UKCC, conducts an investigation. When registered nurses have been found guilty of abuse they are normally struck off the register and can no longer practice.

Preventing abuse

The way a home is managed can make abuse more or less likely to occur. In homes where older people are respected and treated with dignity and respect, the possibility of abuse is reduced. In this atmosphere older people and their families will have developed a good relationship with the manager and staff and will be able to raise concerns. Listening to and communicating with older people individually and at regular patient meetings will help prevent abuse or detect it quickly.

A home where staff are supported and supervised will prevent staff from feeling 'useless', 'out of their depth' and reaching the end of their tether because they are unable to cope with certain situations. A programme of staff education and training helps all staff to develop a greater understanding of the needs of older people. An educational programme helps staff to feel valued, and increased knowledge leads to improved care. In many homes where older people have been neglected the main problem has been that the staff did not know how to meet the needs of older people. In homes where abuse has occurred unchecked, staff morale is poor, many staff have had no training for many years and management has been ineffective.

The home should have a series of procedures in place that help to detect signs of abuse quickly. Each home is required to keep details of accidents – further details are given in Chapter 3. Every accident that occurs should be written in the accident book. If the home has a policy of reviewing accidents and investigating the reasons for them any abuse can be quickly detected, investigated and action taken. A record of any pressure sores that occur will quickly detect cases of poor care and neglect. A record of complaints and suggestions will help detect problems in the early stages.

Financial abuse

Financial abuse can occur. In many homes, the older person keeps a small amount of money with them and money is held by the home for safekeeping. Staff can use this money to buy items such as toiletries or snacks for the residents. It is essential, if the home holds money for the individual's use, that complete records are kept of this. The record should give details of money received and spent. This record protects staff against allegations of financial abuse.

Occasionally relatives who collect the personal allowance for the older person fail to pass this money on to the individual and fail to supply items that the person requires, despite requests from staff. In the past, when fees were met from DSS funds, there was little that could be done in this situation, as the DSS did not wish to be involved. Since the introduction of the Community Care Act, the situation has changed. If staff at the home ask the relative either to purchase items or leave money for these and the relative refuses, social services will act. If the staff suspect that the relative or 'friend' is stealing the personal allowance, this can be discussed with the manager of the home. The manager will discuss the

Name: *Mrs Daisy Brown*

Date	Income/Description	Amount	Outgoings Description	Balance
23/6/99	Pension	£14.75	–	£14.75
27/6/99			Toiletries £3	£11.75
			Chocolate £2.25	£9.50
30/6/99	Pension	£14.75		£24.25
2/7/99			Perm £16	£8.25

Fig. 4.1 Example of record of resident's money.

situation with social services, and social services will investigate and act to ensure that the older person receives a personal allowance.

Abuse from other residents

Residents can abuse other residents in the home. This abuse can take many forms. It ranges from ignoring or 'putting down' an individual, to bullying, theft and physical or sexual abuse. You need to be aware that this can occur and report any suspicions you have to your manager.

Caring for older people who are confused

Older people who are confused may be more at risk of abuse than other residents. Staff may find caring for confused residents less rewarding and more exhausting. This section deals with the causes of confusion and aims to enable you to provide sensitive care to people who are confused. This reduces behavioural problems and the risk of abuse developing.

It is easy to label older people as confused. A few years ago, a nurse who was studying for an elderly care qualification conducted a survey on how older people are treated. She went shopping and got on buses. When she lost her way and asked for help people were helpful. When she misheard, people repeated what they had said. Then, wearing make-up and a wig so that she looked old, she did exactly the same things. People were less helpful and treated her as a confused old lady, not because of her behaviour but because of her age. As adults we are allowed to mishear, mis-understand or be absent minded, but older people who behave in the same way can quickly be labelled as confused.

People who have difficulty in communicating can easily be wrongly labelled as confused. The deaf person who understands only part of the conversation may be thought confused. The person who has suffered a stroke and who uses the wrong word may be thought of as confused. It is important that staff listen to the older person and make sure that the person is not having difficulty in communicating, before deciding that they are confused.

Causes of confusion

Confusion is not a disease, it is a symptom. The first sign of illness in many older people is that they become confused. If this happens, the carer should ask that a professional nurse or doctor sees the patient to find out the cause of the confusion. It can he caused by either physical or mental illness. Many people who become confused will recover if the cause of the confusion is treated, but there is no cure for dementia at present. Causes of confusion include:

- Chest infection
- Urine infection
- Wound infection
- Diabetes
- Anaemia
- An imbalance of chemicals in the blood (electrolyte imbalance)
- Medication
- Head injury
- Thyroid disease – a thyroid gland which is underactive produces less of the hormone thyroxin; a deficiency of this hormone slows the person down physically and mentally
- Parkinson's disease
- Depression
- Dementia
- Dehydration

Treatment of physical causes of confusion

Infection can cause confusion. If the infection is caused by a virus (such as the flu virus), antibiotics will not help. Antibiotics are only effective in treating bacteria. There are two main types of bacteria, known as gram negative and gram positive because of their appearance under the microscope. Certain antibiotics are only effective in treating gram negative or gram positive bacteria. Other antibiotics are effective in treating diseases caused by both gram negative and gram positive bacteria; these are known as broad spectrum antibiotics.

In recent years more of the bacteria that cause infections in older people living in homes have become resistant to the more commonly used antibiotics. If the bacteria are resistant to the antibiotic, the antibiotic will not cure the infection. Many homes now have policies to prevent the spread of infection. These often include sending specimens to ensure that the correct antibiotic is used. The person with a suspected urine infection would have a specimen of urine sent to the microbiology laboratory, where the staff would check for the presence of infection and advise the doctor on the most effective antibiotic to use.

If diabetes is suspected, investigations will be carried out and treatment given. This may include insulin injections or tablets or, if the diabetes is mild, a diabetic diet.

If thyroid disease is present a blood sample will be sent to check the level of thyroid hormone, and tablets containing the hormone thyroxin will be given if required.

If the person is thought to be suffering from Parkinson's disease the doctor will examine them and prescribe medication to treat the disease. This is usually very effective in the early stages of the disease.

If anaemia has caused confusion this will be investigated. Any disease, which has caused the anaemia, will be treated. Iron tablets will normally be prescribed, and the older person will be encouraged to eat a diet rich in iron.

An imbalance in the chemicals in the blood (known as electrolytes) can cause confusion. This imbalance may be caused by medication such as diuretic tablets, diarrhoea, overuse of laxatives or prolonged vomiting. Any imbalance will be treated.

If medication has caused the confusion, the person's doctor will alter the medication. If head injury has caused confusion, urgent hospital treatment will be required. If depression has caused the person to become confused, the doctor may prescribe antidepressant tablets.

Dementia may cause confusion. There is no cure for dementia at present. Dementia is the name used for a group of diseases affecting brain function. There are two main types: multi-infarct dementia and Alzheimer's disease.

Multi-infarct dementia
Multi-infarct dementia is thought to be responsible for 20% of all cases of dementia. A small clot interrupts the blood supply to an area of the brain, and this leads to the death of an area of brain tissue and is known as an infarction. Many of these small infarctions cause brain tissue to die and the person loses the ability to remember and reason.

Multi-infarct dementia is:

■ More common in men, because it is a disease of the arteries supplying the brain. Men are more at risk of arterial disease than women, who are protected from the effects of arterial disease by female hormones that are produced until the menopause. Women of the older generation are less likely to have smoked than men and smoking increases the risk of arterial disease.
■ Often present in people who suffer from high blood pressure (hypertension).
■ Often present in people who have other signs of arterial disease such as angina.

- Sufferers can deteriorate suddenly and then stay at that level until another brain infarction occurs.

Medical treatment aims to prevent or reduce the number of infarcts that will cause brain damage. If the person's blood pressure is high, this will be treated. If the person is overweight, he should be encouraged to lose weight. If he smokes, he should be encouraged to give up. If the person has arterial disease, this will be treated by the doctor. Many people who suffer from multi-infarct dementia are prescribed a junior aspirin each day. Research has shown that this small dose of aspirin helps prevent blood clots forming and greatly reduces the risk of further brain infarction.

Alzheimer's disease

Alzheimer's disease is named after a German neurologist who first described the disease at the beginning of the century. The cause of Alzheimer's disease is not known. There have been many theories over the years but none have been proved. It is known that the number of people suffering from Alzheimer's disease increases with age. Research has shown that 25% of all people over the age of 85 suffer from dementia, and that 80% of those people suffer from Alzheimer's disease.

Alzheimer's disease is a gradual slow deterioration of mental function; memory loss is the first sign. The person has difficulty in learning new things but old memories are retained: the person remembers family but may forget about the new grandchild who was born recently; old skills and habits are retained but the person can easily become lost in new places.

Caring for people suffering from dementia

Dementia is a progressive disease. People who suffer from it have a vast range of abilities. In the early stages of dementia, the individual may be forgetful, have difficulty handling money or remembering what is for lunch. In the advanced stages, the individual may be unable to recognise her daughter or her own face in the mirror. She may be unable to wash, dress, use the toilet, eat independently, or walk without a great deal of help from staff. Obviously, the type of care required is very different, but the aims of care remain the same.

Some people who suffer from dementia cope well because they have a routine. This gives the day structure and they depend on this routine to help them cope. It is important, if a routine is established, that everyone maintains it. If the person normally has breakfast and then bathes, dresses, and has coffee in her room, a change in the routine can cause the person to become confused and disorientated.

The older person should be treated with dignity and respect. Their preferred title should be used. A retired doctor may wish to be referred to as Dr Lawson and a retired headmistress may wish to be known as Miss Anderson. Staff who use first names to address people who have been referred to all their lives by their titles, deprive the older person of dignity and respect and may increase confusion.

It is easy for staff to see all confused older people as lacking in personality and to treat all people with dementia in the same way. Staff should aim to care for the individual. If the person is unable to express preferences, relatives and friends can often tell staff about the person's preferences. The woman who liked to have her hair premed and set should be encouraged and helped to maintain her usual hairstyle. The woman who preferred to wear trousers and blouses should not be discouraged from wearing these clothes because dresses are 'easier'. The person who detests fish and who is unable to request an alternative should have this noted so that she does not refuse lunch and go hungry or spend the afternoon trying to get into the kitchen to find some food. People suffering from dementia are often able to continue to perform activities that they have been doing for decades, such as washing or dressing, although they may forget the way to the dining room. You should aim to provide support and help without taking over and encouraging the person to depend on staff for care before this is required.

If the person enters the home suffering from mild confusion and the early stages of dementia, staff can get to know the person. When the person deteriorates and is unable to communicate needs to staff, this is seldom a problem because staff carers know the person very well. If a person is admitted to the home with advanced dementia, it can be difficult to provide the type of care the person would prefer because staff do not know the person. Relatives and friends can be a great help in these circumstances. They can tell staff what food the person prefers, what her interests are and how she likes to dress and style her hair. In some homes, a written record of this is kept so that all staff can treat the person as she would wish.

Wandering

Some older people wander around the home. This wandering can upset other residents and can make staff feel on edge. Although the older person appears to be wandering around aimlessly, they have a reason for wandering. Unfortunately, not all people suffering from dementia wander for the same reasons. Research has shown that people who wander have great difficulty in communicating their needs. It has been suggested that the person's wandering is an attempt to meet those needs.

Shouting and screaming

You may meet residents who shout, scream, or sing continually. Staff and other residents can find this behaviour difficult to cope with. A great deal can be done to help people who behave like this. You should seek professional advice. Often the person's GP will ask a nurse specialising in psychiatric nursing to see the person. The aim of treatment is first to discover the reasons for the person behaving in this way, and then to plan care to eliminate or reduce such behaviour.

Aggression

Some older people lash out and shout, hit, kick and bite. In many cases the person is confused and may be unaware of your intentions. You should do everything possible to ensure that the older person is aware of what is about to happen, for example: 'Mrs Greendale, I'd like to help you to have a bath now'.

If the person understands what your intentions are and what is happening, aggression is less likely to occur. If the person refuses to bathe, dress or get up, you must not try to force the person. This is unlawful and can lead to aggression. Try leaving the person and returning a little later. The way you approach people is very important. If you have a good relationship with the person and have the right approach, problems are rarer. If a resident becomes aggressive inform your manager.

If a person is aggressive the reasons for the aggression should be determined and care planned to avoid such incidents. Sometimes the older person is extremely aggressive and could injure staff or other residents when lashing out. Residents and staff should not be placed in this situation. If the person is very disturbed, he or she will require care from registered nurses specially trained in caring for people with mental health problems. These nurses are known as Registered Mental Nurses (RMN). This specialist care may be given either in hospital or more usually in a specialist nursing home known as an Elderly Mentally Infirm (EMI) home.

Conclusion

All older people should be treated with dignity and respect.

Caring for older people who are confused, who appear to wander aimlessly, who scream, shout or sing, can be difficult and frustrating. The way that staff handle residents who suffer from dementia influences that person's behaviour. Staff attitudes and care can reduce or increase problems. You may see staff treat people with dementia as if they are children. You may even be told, 'They're just babies really'. Older people with dementia are not babies and are not 'in their second childhood', but are older people suffering from an incurable disease that affects brain function. Treating such people as babies not only denies them the dignity and respect that they deserve, but also worsens problem behaviour and increases the likelihood of abuse.

The likelihood of abuse is increased because staff can come to view residents as less than human. People with dementia can be seen not as people suffering from a dreadful incurable disease, but as objects. If you provide thoughtful sensitive care and ensure that the older person is treated with dignity and respect you will find the older person responds to such care and that problem behaviour is rare.

Abuse in homes is rare. I hope that you never see it. Most staff do a wonderful job of caring for residents. I hope that throughout your career you see people treated with dignity and respect. If you do see abuse occur, you must do something to stop it.

Portfolio preparation

Assessors and students find this unit difficult. Your assessor needs to ensure that you have the skills and knowledge to recognise the indicators of abuse and respond to abuse if you encounter it. Before beginning this module, you should discuss how the assessor intends to assess your skills and knowledge. You may be asked to provide the following types of evidence:

- Witness testimony – this is a statement from a senior member of staff
- Written work reflecting on the difficulties of detecting abuse
- Written work about how you would act if you suspected that abuse was occurring
- Projects about abuse

Your assessor will also use other methods to help you gain evidence for this unit. These may include:

- Verbal questioning about abuse
- Verbal questioning about the home's policy on abuse
- Written questions on abuse
- Simulations

Further information

These are national organisations that provide advice and information.

Action on Elder Abuse
Astral House
1268 London Road
London SW16 4ER
Tel. 020 8679 2468
This charity provides information and leaflets including *Elder Abuse in Care Homes* and *Abuse of Elderly People: Guide-lines for Action*. These are available free of charge (send an SAE).

Age Concern (England)
Astral House
1268 London Road
London SW16 4ER
Tel. 020 8679 8000
Age Concern offers information and advice on nursing and residential home care. They produce a range of leaflets, fact sheets and information.

Alzheimer's Disease Society
Gordon House
10 Greencoat Place
London SW1P 1PH
Tel. 020 7306 0606
This society provides information and advice to relatives and staff who care for people with dementia. They produce a range of free fact sheets, books and a monthly newsletter. They run a series of courses for staff who work with older people suffering from dementia.

Counsel and Care
Twyman House
16 Bonny Street
London NW1 9PG
Tel. 020 7485 1550 for administration and general enquiries. The advice line (staffed from 10 AM to 3.30 PM) is 0845 300 7585. Counsel and Care offer information and advice on nursing and residential home care. They have published a number of books.

Public Concern at Work
Suite 306
16 Baldwin Gardens
London EC1N 7RJ
Tel. 020 7404 6609
Public Concern at Work is a legal advice centre. They offer
information and support.

Further reading

Eastman, M. (ed.) (1995) *Old Age Abuse: A New Perspective*.
    Age Concern and Chapman Hall (co-publishers), London.
Harvey, M. (1990) *Who's confused?* Prepar Publications, Bir-
    mingham.
Hicks, C. (1988) *Who Cares. Looking After Older People at
    Home*. Virago Press, London.
Pritchard, J. (1996) *Working with Elder Abuse*. A training
    manual for home care, residential and day care staff. Jessica
    Kingsley, London.
Stokes, G. (1988) *Wandering*. Winslow Press, Bicester.
Stokes, G. (1988) *Screaming and Shouting*. Winslow Press,
    Bicester.
Tomlin, S. (1988) *Abuse of Elderly People: An Unnecessary
    Problem*. Public information report. British Geriatrics Society,
    London.

Chapter 5

Record Keeping and Confidentiality

Introduction

This chapter covers the option group A units CU5, CU5.1, CU5.2 – 'receive, transmit and store information'. It gives details on how information is collected and stored within the home and how confidentiality is maintained.

This chapter includes:

- ■ Pre-admission assessments
- ■ Legal requirements – which records must be kept
- ■ New National Required Standards
- ■ Care plans and progress notes
- ■ Who writes care plans and progress notes
- ■ Medical records storage and access
- ■ Maintaining confidentiality
- ■ Dealing with relatives
- ■ Telephone enquiries
- ■ Recording details of resident's money
- ■ Caring for valuable and precious items

The importance of communication

Any decision that we make is only as good as the information it is based on. Communication is vitally important to the quality of care. Staff need to communicate effectively if they are to give the best possible care.

As a care assistant, you will work closely with residents. Often the resident will discuss her condition with you. She may say, 'I'm finding it difficult to move around because the pain in my knee is so bad. Those tablets they give me don't seem to be working. But I mustn't grumble or complain. There are lots of people worse off than me'. This information is important. In such situations, you should obtain the person's consent to let senior staff know. Then the GP can be informed and treatment reviewed. Effective communication leads to the resident receiving effective treatment to control pain and improve mobility.

Older people depend on the staff working within homes, and staff have a duty to act in a professional way and protect the confidentiality of information that they gain in the course of their work.

Assessments

Most homes now assess people before admission. An example of a patient assessment sheet is given in Fig. 5.1. Assessments are normally carried out by a senior member of staff. In residential homes, this will be the manager. In nursing homes the matron, deputy matron or a senior RN will carry out the assessment.

The person assessing will visit the older person, who may be living at home, in a residential home (if nursing home admission is being considered) or may be in hospital. The aims of assessment are to meet the older person and to check that the home can meet the individual's care needs. If the manager of a residential home discovers that the older person has nursing needs, the manager may suggest that a nursing home is more appropriate. Under current legislation, residential homes should provide the type of care that would be given by a caring relative at home.

If the older person is extremely confused, with a long history of dementia, and may leave the home and be at risk of being run over on the busy road outside the home, the matron may suggest that the individual requires care in a nursing home registered for the elderly mentally infirm. In such a home the individual would benefit from the care of nurses trained to meet the person's mental health needs.

If the person assessing feels that the home can meet the patient's care needs, the assessment gives both the older person and the member of staff the opportunity to meet and discuss the home. If possible, the older person should visit the home. If the person is recovering from an illness in hospital, this is not always possible and relatives or friends may visit on the person's behalf.

Next time someone from your home is visiting an older person to carry out an assessment, ask if you can go. This will give you an opportunity to watch an assessment and get to know the older person before admission. The information obtained at assessment enables the assessor to begin to plan care.

Patient records

Current legislation requires homes to maintain certain records and sets out how homes should be run. Legislation differs in England,

RESIDENT ASSESSMENT SHEET

Name:	Room Permanent/Temporary
Address:	D.O.B. Age Date/Time admitted:
	Accompanied by:
Tel No:	
Marital Status:	Type of Admission: Emergency Waiting List
Religion:	
Next of Kin:	Reason for Admission:
Relationship:	
Address:	Confirmed Diagnosis:
Tel No:	
Contact in Emergency:	Patient aware of reason for admission:
G.P.	Urinalysis Weight:
Address:	
Tel No:	Past Medial History *(serious illnesses & hospitalisation)*
Lives alone: Yes/No	
Property: *if any valuables are stored, state what and where*	
Discharge/Transfer	
When:	
Where to:	Allergies:
Transport:	
Reason:	
TTAS:	Investigations and Date:
Relatives informed	
General Appearance:	Vision:
Mobility–help needed	Elimination:
Walking Dressing	Urinary:
Bathing Eating	
Comments:	Bowel:
Mental State:	Nutritional State:
Comments:	Dietary Preferences:
	Special Diet:
Skin State:	Sleep:
Broken Areas:	Usual Pattern
Norton Score:	Sedation
Oral Inspection:	Pain–Description:
Dentures Full/Partial	
Hearing:	Leisure Activities, Interests:
Uses Aid	
	History taken by:
	From:

Fig. 5.1   Resident assessment sheet.

Wales, Scotland and Northern Ireland. In all the countries homes are required to keep admission records, records of accidents and a daily record of patient treatment.

Admission records

Homes are required to keep a register of all residents admitted to the home. This should include details of the person's name, address, place admitted from (for example a local hospital), GP's name, the address and telephone numbers of the next of kin, name of person arranging the admission, details of funding and the date of admission. The date of discharge or death should be entered when the patient leaves the home. If the person dies the time and cause of death must be entered.

In residential homes, care assistants normally fill in the admission register. In most nursing homes it is considered the responsibility of registered nurses, although the reasons for this are unclear. In hospitals, the admission register may be filled in by the ward clerk, a care assistant, or a registered nurse. Ask if your home has a policy on who can complete the admission register. Perhaps the registered nurses would welcome help in completing paperwork when a patient is admitted. These records must be retained by law for one year after the last entry. Many homes retain these records for seven years after the last entry.

Daily statements of patient's health

Homes are required by law to keep a daily statement of patient's health. One record of the patient's health must be entered every 24 hours by law. In practice, most homes write in the patient's records twice in 24 hours. One record is normally made by the day staff and one by the night staff.

National required standards

The Registered Homes Acts are both rather old. The government is introducing new legislation. The Care Standards Bill 2000 is expected to become law by summer 2000 and is expected to be enacted in stages. It introduces new national required standards. These are minimum standards that each home must meet. At the time of writing the standards have been drawn up and released as a consultation document. It appears that the standards would be implemented in 2001 at the earliest. The draft of these new standards specifies the type of records homes would be required to keep. The current legislation does not specify how records are to be kept.

Care plans

In the past, patient care was planned based on 'task allocation'. Each member of the team was allocated tasks that took account of the abilities of that member of staff. One member of staff might have been asked to check all the patients' temperatures, pulses and blood pressures. Another two members of staff might have been asked to make all the beds. This system of care had several drawbacks. The first was that residents were cared for by many different staff and few residents got to know staff. Also, staff felt as if they were working on a production line and that they had little opportunity to get to know residents. Using a task allocation system meant that most residents with the same condition were treated in exactly the same way.

The system now used in most homes is that of individualised patient care. This aims to treat the person as an individual. Two people who have arthritis in the knees may have entirely different priorities and needs. Mrs Cain, for example, may have difficulty in walking because of her arthritis and this may be preventing her from attending church on Sundays. Mr Edwards may find that the pain in his knees is preventing him from getting a good night's sleep.

The basis of individualised care is the care plan. This plan is drawn up in consultation with the patient. In nursing homes trained nurses use a 'nursing model' to help them draw up the care plan. There are a number of nursing models and one commonly used was drawn up by Roper, Logan and Tierney (1990). This model identifies twelve activities of daily living (Fig. 5.2). The nurse uses these activities to help plan care.

The care plan is used to identify the patient's needs, the aims of nursing care, the action that is taken to help meet these needs and the outcome of the care. A copy of a care plan is shown in Fig. 5.3.

Information recorded on a care plan

The care plan contains information about the person's day to day care.

It should give details of any assistance required to wash or bathe; this may include using a bath hoist. It will also include the person's preferences, for example if the person prefers to bath or shower.

It should give details of the person's mobility. If the person uses a frame to walk this should be recorded. If the person requires a walking aid and the help of one or two members of staff to walk, this will be recorded.

If the person has a continence problem, this should be recorded. A separate continence assessment will also have been undertaken

1. Maintaining a safe environment
2. Communication
3. Breathing
4. Eating and drinking
5. Eliminating
6. Personal cleansing and dressing
7. Controlling body temperature
8. Mobilizing
9. Sleeping
10. Religious needs
11. Social activity
12. Expressing sexuality
13. Wounds and dressings
14. Dying

The nurse may identify other needs.

Fig. 5.2 Activities of daily living (Roper, Logan & Tierney 1990).

and this will be kept separately. Treatment to promote continence such as a toileting programme or bladder retraining will be noted on the care plan.

If the older person requires a special diet, has difficulty in feeding herself, or requires aids to enable her to eat independently, this will be noted on the care plan.

The care plan should identify the person's needs and the aims of care, and give details of how that care is to be given. After a time, the effectiveness of the care given will be evaluated.

Care assistants should read the older person's care plan so that they are aware of the care required and the reasons that this particular care is given. A care assistant might think that it is cruel to expect a person who has recently had surgery to repair a fractured femur to begin walking again. The care plan should explain the reasons why the older person should be encouraged to walk again.

Care assistants can often help trained staff give better care by informing them of how the person is feeling. The individual may tell you that pain is making it difficult for her to walk but she does not want to 'bother' the nurse. If you find out and inform the nurse, arrangements can be made to ensure that the patient receives satisfactory pain relief. In this way nurses and care assistants can work together to ensure that the older person receives care of the highest quality.

Sometimes trained nurses use technical terms that you may not

Date	Needs	Aim	Action	Evaluation
23/6/99	To keep	To help	1) Walk with Mrs Morris	
	clean and	Mrs Morris	to bathroom	
①	fresh	bathe and	2) Use hoist to help her	
		wash	get into bath	
			3) Help Mrs Morris wash	
			her back and feet	
			4) Leave Mrs Morris to	
			soak if she wishes	
			5) Ensure Mrs Morris	
			can reach call bell	
②	To walk	1) To help	1) Help to put caliper	
	independently	Mrs Morris	on left leg	
		remain able	2) Assist with putting	
		to walk	on shoes	
		independently	3) Ensure Mrs Morris's	
			tripod is within easy	
			reach	

Name: Mrs Edna Morris   Room No: 2   Age: 92

Fig. 5.3 Sample care plan.

understand. In this book, all technical terms used are explained. Nursing staff sometimes use abbreviations and initials and these can appear confusing to care assistants. You can look these up in the glossary. The United Kingdom Central Council, the body responsible for regulating nurses, recommends that nurses do not use abbreviations and initials in nursing records. Abbreviations are confusing and can lead to error. If you do not understand terms or see abbreviations used in nursing records, ask the nursing staff to explain. They will usually be pleased to do so and will be delighted that you are keen to learn.

Progress report

A progress report (Fig. 5.4) is used as a daily record of the individual's care. The information recorded in the progress notes goes from home to home. Check the policy in your home about what is recorded in the patient's progress notes.

Progress report

Date & time	Progress	Signature
23/6/99	Bathed with help. Hair set and dressed in new blue dress and jacket.	
Day	Daughter visited at 2pm with family to celebrate Mr & Mrs Morris's diamond wedding anniversary.	N Davis
Night	Settled late but had a wonderful day. Looking forward to seeing pictures that family took.	L Dominguez
Name Mrs Edna Morris	Room 4	Date of birth 17/11/11

Fig. 5.4 Sample of a progress report.

Who writes care plans and progress notes?

Some residential homes now employ registered nurses. Although under the terms of legislation RNs are not to use their nursing skills in residential homes, in practice many do. If the residential home you are working in employs a registered nurse or a number of registered nurses they may write the care plans and progress notes. In residential homes where registered nurses are not employed, care assistants will be responsible for writing care plans and maintaining progress notes. These will be less detailed than those kept by nursing homes because the people living in residential homes do not require nursing care.

If a person living in a residential home is being visited by a district nurse, perhaps to treat a leg ulcer, the district nurse may write in the care plan. If the person is receiving therapy from another professional, such as speech therapy, the speech therapist may wish to write in the care plan. The speech therapist may write instructions and advice that help you enable the person to make progress with speech between treatments. The policy will vary from home to home. Find out what the policy is in your home.

In nursing homes, the policy will also vary from home to home. In large homes that have several registered nurses on each shift, all records may be kept by registered nurses. The registered nurse writing the report will normally discuss the care of any patient with the care assistant who has given the care. The registered nurse will then complete the report. If you are aware of any changes in the person's condition or if the older person has told you something that the registered nurse may not be aware of you should inform the registered nurse.

You may be helping the individual to get up after an afternoon nap and notice that the person appears pale and faint. You should inform the registered nurse or your manager. The reasons for this can be investigated and further action taken.

In some homes, care assistants may be asked to fill in the progress reports. Any entry is checked by the registered nurse, who countersigns the entry. In this situation care assistants should be instructed and helped to fill in such reports by the registered nurse or manager. Check the procedure in your home. In nursing homes other professionals such as physiotherapists, speech therapists, nurses specialising in the care of people with diabetes, or continence advisers will be frequent visitors. This is because older people who live in nursing homes require greater levels of skilled care than those living in residential homes. In many homes, these professionals will write in the care plan.

Further records stored in the home

People living in homes have other records. When the older person is admitted to the home, a letter is normally sent from the person's GP if the person was admitted from their own home. If the person was admitted from hospital, a note will have been sent to the home. If the person's GP has asked other professionals, such as a physiotherapist, speech therapist or clinical nurse specialist, to treat the patient, a referral letter will be written. Details of inpatient visits while the person is living in the home will also need to be stored. Old care plans, medication charts and other papers will require storage. In many homes, each resident has a folder containing all records. Many GPs also write notes about the treatment they prescribe and keep them in this folder. Although GPs keep separate records detailing patient treatment, they may also keep notes at the home. GPs prefer to do this in case the patient needs to be seen by another doctor in an emergency or patient records are required by hospital staff. These records are normally stored in a locked cupboard or filing cabinet in the home, to protect confidentiality.

Computerised records

Some homes are now using computers to plan and manage care and to keep records. If computerised records are used in your home, you will receive training to enable you to use the system. Some homes use electronic mail (e-mail) to send information from one home to another. If the home you work in uses e mail, you can ask how to use this.

Facsimile transmissions

Sending information by a facsimile is now common place. If there is a fax machine in your home find out the policy for communicating information received in facsimiles and how facsimile information is filed.

Access to medical and nursing records

Residents now have a legal right to have access to their health records under the Access to Medical Records Act which became law in 1990. The patient writes to the doctor who is providing care, normally the older person's GP in homes, and requests copies of all records.

Nursing homes are inspected by registration and inspection officers employed by the local NHS trust. Residential homes are inspected by inspection officers employed by social services. Inspection officers have the power to ask to see day to day records relating to care. They do not have the right to see medical records unless the inspector is a qualified medical practitioner. The government have now announced plans to merge the nursing and residential home inspectorates into an independent inspection unit. Inspection units will be divided into regions.

Confidentiality

Staff who work with older people learn a great deal about those they care for. All staff must ensure that information that they discover in the course of their work remains confidential. Most care assistants are very aware of how essential it is to maintain confidentiality at all times; however, staff can inadvertently betray confidentiality. This may occur in the following situations:

- Discussing the patient's condition with another member of staff within earshot of other residents or relatives
- In conversation outside of work, perhaps at the bus stop, on a train or in a restaurant or pub, where this conversation may be overheard by others
- By using the patient's name in NVQ evidence gathering – normally initials are used to maintain confidentiality
- By leaving patient records lying around – the nursing notes or other records may be left where other residents have access to them
- By disclosing information about the person's condition to relatives and friends without their consent.

It is important that care assistants are always aware of the need to maintain confidentiality, as the relationship between care assistant and patient is built on trust. Betraying that trust may destroy the caring relationship.

Dealing with relatives

Many relatives will approach care assistants, even junior members of staff who have not been working in the home for very long, and ask how the patient is. It is important that you find out the home's policy on giving information to relatives. Care assistants who have worked in hospital before may have been told to refer all queries to registered nurses. In many homes, the policy will be different. In most homes, the enquiry is partly a way of starting a conversation with the care assistant and only a general answer is required. For example, Mrs Jenkin's daughter might say:
'Hello Julie, I've come to see Mum. How is she today?'

In this case, the care assistant would reply, 'Well, she's just had her hair done and she's been looking forward to your visit.'

In other cases the relative might be asking for more specific information, but the care assistant can deal with this; for example, Mrs Franklin's daughter asks:
'How did mum get on at the opticians when she had her eyes tested?'

The care assistant might reply, 'The optician said she needs new glasses so she's chosen the frames and they should be ready on Tuesday.'

In other cases the care assistant may not have the information or may not be able to answer the relative's questions fully and should ask the registered nurse or the home's manager to speak to the relative; for example, Mrs Davis' daughter asks:
'How did mum get on down at the hospital when she saw the specialist about her arthritic hip?'

The care assistant might reply, 'I think the specialist spoke to Sister James about her hip. If you hold on I'll just see if I can find her and she can have a word with you.'

In each of these examples the care assistant has given the relative as much information and help as possible. The care assistant has shown the relative that she is aware of the patient's treatment but is not getting out of her depth and attempting to give information which she does not completely understand.

Telephone queries

In many homes, the matron or manager answers the telephone whenever possible and deals with telephone queries. When the person in charge is busy, other staff often answer the telephone. It is important to state the name of the home and your name when answering, for example 'High Trees Nursing Home, Penny Jones speaking,' or 'care assistant Jones speaking'. This helps maintain the home's professional image. Always find out who is calling, and if the person is asking to speak to the person in charge ask the nature of their call. If the nurse in charge of the nursing home is attending to a patient who is ill and she is aware that the call is from the representative of a company selling cleaning products, she can give you a message to tell them to call back at a more convenient time. Many relatives and friends telephone to ask how residents are. This is often just a general enquiry, for example:

'This is Mrs Gibson. How is my mum, Mrs Kelly, today?'

'She's fine; all her birthday cards have arrived and she's opening them now.'

'Can you tell her we'll pick her up at 1 o'clock and take her out to lunch?'

If Mrs Kelly was unwell, the care assistant would fetch the person in charge who could speak to the relative.

Many homes have a policy about who should answer the telephone, who should give certain information and under what circumstances this information is given. Many homes do not tell relatives over the telephone that a person has died, unless the older person has been ill and the death is expected. Find out policies in your home on relaying information over the telephone. If you are unsure of what to say in certain circumstances ask a more senior member of staff to take the call.

Caring for the older person's possessions

People living in homes may ask staff to look after possessions for them. The home should have a policy on looking after money and valuables for residents. Some older people ask their families to look after possessions, while others prefer to leave these at home. Some older people living in homes do not have any family and friends and rely on staff to help them look after possessions. Older people living in homes whose fees are paid by either social services under the Community Care Act 1993 or who have their fees met by the Department of Social Security (DSS) under earlier funding arrangements, are entitled to a 'personal allowance'. This allowance is £15.45 per week, as at April 2000, and is to enable older people to buy clothing and other items that they may require.

Keeping records of residents' money

Homes are obliged to keep a record of any money that they look after for older people. In many homes residents ask staff to buy things for them at the shops. Whenever possible older people should be encouraged to accompany staff to the shops and given the opportunity to select and buy things themselves. When staff buy things for residents a full record of the money spent should be kept. This protects residents from financial abuse and protects staff from any accusations of theft. An example of such a record is given in Chapter 4 (Fig. 4.1)

Keeping records of other items left for safekeeping

Staff may be asked to keep other items for the patient. A record of this should be kept. This may be a note in the patient's progress notes or it may be written in a book kept for this purpose, normally known as a property or valuables book. Care assistants should be careful about recording items. All that glitters is not gold and all white stones that sparkle are not diamonds. You should record 'one yellow metal ring with a white stone' not 'gold ring with diamond solitaire'.

Residents who retain valuable items

Some older people wear valuable items and do not wish to leave them in the home's safe. They have every right to continue to wear valuable items of jewellery. Imagine how you would feel if your treasured engagement ring or locket was taken away and locked in a safe in case you lose it. If the older person is wearing rings or has brought jewellery into the home a note of this should be made. Many homes state that they cannot take responsibility for items that have been lost unless a robbery has taken place. In some homes, residents can take out an insurance policy to insure against losing valuables.

It is important that relatives and staff communicate well. Staff in countless homes have spent hours searching for 'lost' rings only to discover later that relatives have taken them to jewellers to have them adjusted because they no longer fit. In the home where I worked, several staff spent hours searching for a ring that a for-getful patient had misplaced. We found the ring finally in the dustbag in the vacuum cleaner. Later we discovered that the ring we thought we were searching for, which had been in the older person's family for over a hundred years, had in fact been replaced with a copy by the patient's family with her consent. The patient had forgotten to tell us and so had the relatives.

Precious items

Some items such as spectacles, hearing aids and dentures have no value to anyone except their owner. You can help residents to keep track of such possessions. If such items are lost and cannot be found, replacements should be organised. Spectacles can be engraved with the owner's surname or initials by many opticians. The person who is in the habit of taking off reading glasses and putting them down might like to wear a chain. These chains attach to the arms of the glasses and when the person is not reading the glasses can be folded down and can rest on the chest. Some people find these a boon while others detest them; be guided by the individual's wishes. Some people have reading glasses and glasses for distance vision. Bifocal lenses can be used for both reading and distance vision but some people prefer to have two different types of glasses. Encourage people who are having two pairs of glasses to choose different frames for each. This prevents mix-ups. Record descriptions of the glasses in the care plan, for example: 'reading glasses have pink plastic frames; ordinary glasses have gold metal frames'. The optician can also engrave an R, for reading, or a D for distance on the arms of new glasses. Dentures and hearing aids can also be engraved with the person's name if required. Homes can obtain denture-marking kits from the local dentist. Marking can be done discreetly and enables staff to identify possessions that have been misplaced.

Summary

Homes store a variety of records relating to the medical and nursing care of the older people living in the home. Some of this information is extremely sensitive and disclosure could cause great embarrassment to the older person and could breach the caring relationship between staff and patient. Records should be stored in a safe place and only staff should have access to these records. The older person has the legal right to see these records on request. Older people grow to respect and trust their care assistants. Care assistants have a duty to ensure that patient confidentiality is maintained at all times.

Portfolio preparation

This unit aims to assess your ability to receive, transmit, store and retrieve information. Assessors will use a variety of strategies to assess your ability to meet the standards specified. Before beginning this module, discuss assessment strategies with your assessor. Most of this unit can be assessed using direct observation. You may be asked to provide the following types of evidence:

- Products. This might include a copy of patient records that you have completed. Remember to delete the resident's name to preserve confidentiality.
- Witness testimony – a statement from a senior member of staff.
- Written work – you might be asked to prepare an A4 sheet on how to ensure that you maintain confidentiality.

Your assessor will also use other methods to help you gain evidence for this unit. These may include:

- Verbal questioning
- Written questions

Simulations are not considered a suitable assessment method for this unit.

Further information

Access to Health Records Act 1990. The Stationery Office, London. Your local college may have a copy of this Act in the library. If not you can visit the reference library at your local library, read the Act and take photocopies if you wish.

References

Roper, Logan & Tierney (1990) *The Elements of Nursing*, 3rd edn. Churchill-Livingstone, Edinburgh.

Chapter 6

Food and Drink

Introduction

This chapter covers the option group A units NC12, NC12.1 and NC12.2 – 'enable clients to eat and drink'; and the option group B units NC13, NC13.1 and NC13.2 – 'prepare food and drink for clients'.

Food and fluids are more than just fuel for our bodies. Meal times can be relaxed pleasurable occasions.

This chapter gives information on:

- The importance of fluids
- Why some older people are at risk of becoming dehydrated
- Normal fluid requirements
- Helping and encouraging patients to drink
- Recording fluid intake and output
- The importance of a healthy diet
- Calories requirements
- What is a healthy diet
- Vitamins and minerals
- Special diets
- Meeting the dietary needs of people from different cultures
- Dietary supplements

The importance of fluids

Healthy people will die within three days if they do not have fluids. Fluid is essential to life. The human body is mostly water in healthy young adults. Women's bodies contain less fluid than men's because women carry more fat on their bodies and fat contains little fluid. The amount of fluid in the body lessens with age. The average older man's body is 55% fluid and the average older woman's body is 45% fluid.

Each day we lose fluid and if the fluid lost is not replaced the amount of fluid in the body is reduced. This process is known as dehydration. Each day the average person loses fluid in:

- Urine – normally 1500 ml is produced
- Breath – normally 400 ml of fluid is lost in the breath
- Faeces – normally 100ml of fluid is lost in faeces
- Sweat – the amount of fluid lost in sweat will vary according to the temperature and how much the individual perspires.

It is important that the individual drinks enough fluid to replace fluids lost by the body. If the person does not drink sufficient fluids, the balance of chemicals (known as electrolytes) within the body is disturbed and this can lead to illness. People who do not drink enough are at risk of developing urine infections. They are more likely to become constipated, have less resistance to infection, and are at risk of developing infections, such as a chest infection, which can lead to serious ill health or even death.

Individuals who become dehydrated may become confused. Dehydration causes the blood to thicken and become more sticky (viscous). The blood is more likely to clot and blood clots can lead to strokes, heart attacks and blood clots in the legs (deep vein thrombosis). All of these can cause serious illness that can lead to the older person becoming more disabled. In some cases, the older person may die because of the complications of dehydration.

Why older people living in homes may become dehydrated

Normally when it is hot or we are in danger of becoming dehydrated we become thirsty. Drinking restores the body's normal fluid balance. This is known as the thirst mechanism. As people age the thirst mechanism becomes less efficient and even when older people are becoming dehydrated they do not feel as thirsty as younger people do. In hot weather or when we are in danger of becoming dehydrated, our kidneys respond by trying to conserve water. Less urine is produced. As people age the kidneys become less efficient at concentrating urine and conserving water.

Some people who live in nursing homes have problems communicating. Even if they are thirsty, they may have difficulty in asking staff for a drink. Some older people living in homes suffer from confusion and although they are thirsty, they may have difficulty in understanding that this is the problem. Confusion gets worse if the individual does not have enough fluid. These individuals depend on staff to leave a drink where they can reach it, perhaps on the patient's locker or table.

Some people are unable to manage to drink without help even if the drink is placed in front of them. People suffering from arthritis may be unable to hold or lift the cup. People with a tremor may drop the cup or glass. The person who has had a stroke or who has poor eyesight may be unable to see the glass.

Some people are reluctant to drink because they suffer from urinary incontinence and are afraid that they will have an accident if they drink. Some people have difficulty in swallowing because illness makes it difficult. People who have had strokes or have Parkinson's disease or motor neurone disease may have difficulty in swallowing. The older person may not like the drink she has been given.

Some individuals may need more fluid than others. A person who has diabetes may pass much more urine than normal. The reasons for this are given later in the chapter. The person may have a leg ulcer or pressure sore that can weep fluid and increase their fluid requirements. The older person may be vomiting, may have diarrhoea, or may feel sick, perhaps because of the medication they are taking, or perhaps because of constipation.

How much fluid do older people normally require?

Older people normally require two litres of fluids each day. Check how much fluid a teacup holds in your home. The average teacup holds approximately 250 ml, but the cups in your home may be slightly larger or smaller than average. Remember when measuring how much a cup holds, that cups are not normally filled to the brim and most people do not drain their cups. Usually a little tea or coffee is left in the bottom of the cup. Check how much fluid the drinking glasses used in your home hold. The capacity of a drinking glass varies more than that of teacups. Drinking glasses hold between 250 and 330 ml on average.

When do older people require extra fluids?

While most people require two litres of fluid each day there are times when individuals require more fluid. If it is hot individuals will sweat more and will require extra fluid to prevent dehydration. Recent research carried out in a Swedish nursing home found that residents liked to spend most of their day in the sunny conservatory. The sun raised the temperature and people who spent most of the day in the conservatory required an extra 500 ml of fluid a day because of increased fluid loss.

When people have an infection, the body fights it by raising the body temperature, because bacteria and viruses are usually killed by higher than normal body temperatures. When the body temperature rises the individual will sweat more and increased fluids are required to replace fluid lost in this way.

Normally approximately 100 ml of fluid is lost in faeces each day. If the older person has diarrhoea, the amount of fluid lost from the bowel increases. Extra fluid is needed to replace this lost fluid. Some older people have had surgery and a piece of small or large bowel is brought to the surface of the abdomen. This opening is known as a stoma. Faeces are collected in a bag that is attached to the abdominal wall. One of the functions of the large bowel (which is known as the colon) is to reabsorb water from faeces. People who have stomas may have either ileostomies (where the small bowel – known as the ileum – is brought to the surface of the abdomen) or colostomies (where a piece of the large bowel is brought to the surface of the abdomen). People who have stomas lose more fluid in their faeces than normal. People who have ileostomies tend to lose much more fluid than those who have colostomies. Individuals who are losing more fluid than average in their faeces must drink extra fluids to make up for the loss.

Older people, especially women, are more likely to develop cystitis and urine infections. These are normally treated with antibiotics but an important part of treating urine infections is encouraging the individual to drink lots of fluid. This helps flush the infection out of the system.

Normally healthy people breathe in and out through the nose. The breathing rate (known as the respiration rate) varies from 12 to 20 times per minute in healthy adults. If the older person develops a heavy cold or a chest infection, the nose can become blocked and the individual breathes through the mouth. The mouth then becomes dry and the amount of fluid lost in breathing is increased. The respiration rate increases when an individual develops a chest infection and the amount of fluid lost in breathing increases. A high temperature will normally develop and this will lead to increased sweating and more fluid will be required.

Helping and encouraging older people to drink

Before you can encourage the older person to drink you need to find out what fluids the individual prefers. There is no point in offering the individual tea four times each day if she detests tea and relishes coffee. Does the person like tea? Does she like it black, with lemon, strong or weak? If the older person prefers sweet tea and cannot have sugar because she has diabetes, it is worth checking which sweetener is preferred. Some can leave a bitter after-taste. If the individual likes sugar in her tea, don't forget to stir the tea or provide a teaspoon, otherwise all the sugar stays in the bottom of the cup, the tea tastes bitter, and the person may not drink it.

If the individual likes coffee find out how she likes it. She may not appreciate mellow powdered coffee and may long for a rich, darkly roasted coffee. On the other hand, she may detest the pungent, almost black coffee offered and prefer coffee made with milk and two sugars.

What cold drinks does the person prefer? Not everyone likes orange squash. Some people may prefer orange barley water, fresh orange juice, lime juice, blackcurrant squash, apple juice or fruits of the forest. Some people may prefer fizzy drinks and may like lemonade, ginger beer, cola or even fizzy water. Low calorie still and fizzy drinks are available for people who are diabetic or who are trying to lose a little weight.

The individual may like to have a can of beer in the evening. You should check with professional staff before suggesting that the older person can have alcohol as some medicines react with alcohol and increase the risk of unpleasant side effects.

Drinks should be served at the right temperature. Orange squash made with cold water is much more appealing than squash made with lukewarm water. Squashes should not be overdiluted as they then look unappealing and have no taste at all. Tea and coffee should be served hot, not lukewarm. You should make sure that tea and coffee is not so hot that it could burn the mouth of a confused patient, or scald someone who accidentally spills the drink onto his or her lap.

If the older person has difficulty in communicating or is confused, family and friends can often advise staff on the individual's preferences. These preferences should be recorded so that all staff can offer preferred fluids.

Some older people may not drink because staff have left a jug of orange but not brought a glass. Sometimes staff are aware that the person does not have a drinking glass and mean to bring it later but forget. Many older people worry about being thought of as 'a nuisance' and do not wish to 'trouble the staff when they are busy'. If the older person does not have a glass, she may remain thirsty for hours. Sometimes the drink is left just out of the older person's reach. Some older people can become forgetful and may forget to have the drink that has been poured and left; popping back to remind the older person only takes a moment and can prevent dehydration. Some older people cannot manage to lift heavy pottery cups full of tea. Providing lightweight cups such as those used on picnics can mean that the individual can drink independently. These cups look and feel just like normal cups. The person or her family could choose lightweight cups if the home does not provide them.

It is almost impossible to drink if you are slumped in a chair or lying in bed. It is important to help the older person sit up comfortably so that she is able to drink. Some residents may have problems swallowing, especially those who have suffered from strokes or who have Parkinson's disease or motor neurone disease. Many of these individuals will require help to sit up and drink. If a person appears to be choking on a drink you should stop giving the drink immediately and seek professional advice. Details of how to cope in an emergency are given in Chapter 3.

Helping frail people to drink

Some older people are unable to drink fluids and rely on staff to give fluids. In many homes, it is assumed that if the person requires help a feeding cup should be used. Feeding cups are usually made of opaque white plastic and have a top with a spout on them.

Many older people can manage to drink from a normal cup if the care assistant holds it to the patient's lips. It is important not to fill the cup too full and to take time helping the person to drink. Some older people manage to drink cold fluids more easily using a flexible straw that bends over. If this is not possible, the care assistant may have no choice but to use a feeding cup, but these should not be used if there is an alternative. Feeding cups give patients very little control over how fast they drink. It can be easy to give the person mouthfuls that are too large to swallow comfortably. Ask one of your colleagues to give you some tea from a teacup. Now ask to be given tea in a feeding cup. Did you feel more in control when drinking from the cup? Which drink was more enjoyable?

You must always remember to offer frail older people the fluids they prefer. Some people do not like to drink a great deal of fluid at once. The care assistant should respect the older person's wishes and offer 'little and often' in such a situation.

Recording fluid intake and output

Sometimes senior staff may decide that an individual's fluid intake and output should be recorded. There are a number of reasons for this. Staff may be unsure how much the individual is drinking. Recording the amount allows staff to check if the person is drinking enough. Sometimes an individual is not drinking enough and all staff are asked to encourage and help the person to have sufficient fluids. The chart allows staff to check how successful they are in giving the person fluids. In other cases staff may be interested in how often the person is passing urine and how much is passed. This information is used to help people who have problems with incontinence. Further details on this are given in Chapter 13. Fluid charts are also called fluid balance charts; an example is given in Fig. 6.1.

Fluid Balance Chart

Name _____ Date _____

Time	Fluid type/amount	R/T	Output type/amount	R/T
	Total intake =		Total output =	

Fig. 6.1 Fluid balance chart.

Fluid charts are normally commenced at midnight. Some have continuous or running totals whilst others are added up at midnight. All fluid taken into the body is recorded on the left-hand side of the chart. This includes fluid given by an intravenous or subcutaneous infusion (drip) or directly into the stomach using either a tube that goes from the patient's nose (nasogastric tube) or one that is stitched into the patient's stomach (gastrostomy tube). Registered nurses in nursing homes will record fluids given intravenously, subcutaneosly or via gastrostomy or nasogastric tubes. Residential homes do not care for older people who require fluids given by these methods.

The right-hand side of the chart is used to record fluids that leave the body. Urine is measured and recorded. If the person vomits the amount of vomit is usually estimated and recorded on this side of the chart. It is important to record fluids as accurately as possible. You may be asked to record fluids which patients have drunk on the fluid balance chart. Senior staff will show you how to do this.

The importance of a healthy diet

Older people require the same amount of vitamins and nutrients as younger people, according to Department of Health guidance. On average, though, older people require fewer calories than younger, more active people. Food provided to older people living in homes needs to be carefully selected. It should be as full of vitamins and nutrients as possible but should have fewer calories than our normal diet. A healthy diet makes the person feel well and protects against infection and illness.

How many calories does an older person require?

The amount of calories required varies from person to person. The active, older person living in a residential home, who is independent, will normally require more calories than the person living in a nursing home who is not active. The less active person living in a nursing home may, however, sometimes require more calories than the average older person. If the person is recovering from a major operation, such as repair of a fractured femur, a diet high in calories, protein and vitamins will be required. If the person has a wound, for example a pressure sore, extra calories, vitamins and protein are required in order to enable the wound to heal.

Some people living in homes will require large portions of food to meet their requirements, whilst others must avoid eating too much if they are to avoid gaining a great deal of weight. Weighing individuals from time to time will warn staff if the person is not having enough food or is gaining weight rapidly. In many hospitals, all elderly people are weighed each week. If the older person is not seriously undernourished, monthly weighings are adequate.

What is a healthy diet?

Over the years, experts have given different and contradictory advice about a healthy diet. No doubt this advice will change again as experts learn more about nutrition. The Department of Health issues dietary guidelines for healthy eating, but these do not apply to elderly people. The guidelines, for example, recommend that adults should drink skimmed milk instead of whole milk, should reduce the amount of fat in their diets, should eat only two or three eggs per week, and should eat cheeses low in fat instead of high fat cheeses such as cheddar. But these recommendations are not suitable for elderly people, who require a diet full of vitamins and nutrients and containing a balance of protein, fat and carbohydrate.

Protein
Protein is found in meat, fish, nuts, lentils and beans. Protein is required to repair and replace tissues. People who have wounds, who have had recent surgery or who are recovering from a major illness require higher than normal amounts of protein.

Carbohydrate
Carbohydrate is found in vegetables and cereals. Carbohydrate is

required to provide energy. It is converted by the body into glucose. Glucose is the body's main source of energy and is required by every living cell.

Fat

Fat is found in meat, fish, nuts, butter, margarine, cheese, eggs and cream. Fat is required to provide energy.

Vitamins and minerals

All food contains vitamins and minerals. Each vitamin and mineral has a function, and a shortage of vitamins or minerals can lead to illness. Some minerals and vitamins are found in most food, and shortage is rare. Others are only contained in a limited range of foods and if the individual does not eat these foods, she may lack these vitamins or minerals.

The minerals and salts required by the body are given below.

Calcium

Calcium is found in milk, butter, cheese and other foods. Calcium is required to maintain healthy teeth and bones. It also affects blood clotting and enables nerve cells to pass messages to each other. Older people can become short of calcium because they do not eat enough dairy produce. Vitamin D is required to enable the body to absorb calcium.

Copper and cobalt

Shortage of these minerals is very rare.

Iodine

Iodine is normally contained in the soil and vegetables grown in such soil absorb it. Sea fish and shellfish are a rich source of iodine.

Most people living in homes eat sea fish at least once a week and are not at risk of iodine deficiency. Even those who do not eat fish get enough iodine from fruit and vegetables.

Iron

Iron is found in red meat, beef, spinach, broccoli, baked beans, apricots and chocolate. Many older people suffer from iron deficiency. This may be because they find it difficult to chew red meat, because they do not eat enough foods containing iron or because they have lost blood following an operation.

Some tablets, especially those given to people who suffer from arthritis – the anti-inflammatory drugs – can irritate the lining of the stomach and bowel. This irritation can cause the stomach and bowel to bleed a little, and this slow bleeding can cause the older person to develop anaemia. Iron tablets are usually given to treat anaemia. Only one tenth of iron in the diet or given in tablet form is normally absorbed by the body. If the person is anaemic, the body absorbs more of the iron given. It has been found that the body can absorb more iron if vitamin C is given at the same time. Giving the older person an orange to eat or a glass of orange juice after iron tablets helps the body to absorb the iron.

Magnesium
Lack of magnesium is rare.

Sodium
This is normal salt. Fruit and vegetables contain salt. Processed foods usually have salt added. Most people add salt to their food and a shortage of salt is rare in this country. In tropical countries individuals may need to take extra salt on their food if they are working very hard and losing salt in their sweat.

Phosphorus
Phosphorus is found in milk, eggs and butter. It is needed to help muscles work properly, to form bones, and to balance the chemicals in the body known as electrolytes. Shortage is very rare.

Zinc
This mineral is required to allow wounds and bones to heal. It is found in liver, eggs, meat and bran. Research in recent years has shown that some people who have wounds that fail to heal, such as pressure sores and leg ulcers, benefit from zinc supplements.

Vitamin A
Vitamin A is found in milk, butter, cream, eggs, liver, carrots and spinach. It is added to margarine. It is required to keep the skin and eyes healthy. Recent research suggests that vitamin A helps to protect the body against developing cancer.

Vitamin B
Vitamin B complex is really a series of vitamins.

Folic acid is found in green leafy vegetables, liver, yeast, Marmite (which is made from yeast) and beer. Shortage of folic acid causes anaemia. Some people who are suffering from anaemia are treated with a mixture of iron (ferrous sulphate) and folic acid.

Niacin is found in cereals, wheat, liver, yeast and fish. Deficiency is usually only found in countries where wheat flour is not eaten, but it can occur in alcoholics. Deficiency causes a disease known as pellagra and the person affected suffers from confusion, dementia, diarrhoea and dermatitis. Pellagra is very rare in the UK.

Thiamine is found in eggs, peas, beans, nuts, yeast, liver, kidneys and the outer husk of rice. Deficiency leads to a disease known as beri beri. It is very rare in the UK as thiamine is found in such a variety of foods.

Riboflavin is found in green vegetables, milk, cheese, eggs, yeast and liver. It is needed to maintain a healthy skin. Deficiency is rare and normally only occurs in people who for medical reasons have been taking antibiotics for a long period.

Vitamin B_{12} is found in meat, especially liver and kidneys. Deficiency causes a special type of anaemia known as pernicious anaemia. Some people are unable to absorb vitamin B_{12} because their stomach lacks a substance necessary to absorb it. People who suffer from vitamin B_{12} deficiency have injections of this vitamin, given monthly or less frequently. Vegetarians can suffer from a shortage of vitamin B_{12} but eating foods containing yeast, such as Marmite, or drinking beer (in moderation) can prevent this.

Vitamin C

Vitamin C is required to maintain a healthy skin and to enable wounds to heal. It is thought that vitamin C protects the body against infection. Fresh fruit and vegetables contain vitamin C. Citrus fruits are high in vitamin C, while apples, pears and plums contain only small amounts. Vitamin C is easily destroyed by cooking, and keeping vegetables warm (for example in a hot trolley) destroys the vitamin C content. Liquidising or puréeing food reduces the vitamin C content.

Vitamin D

Vitamin D is required to produce and maintain strong bones. Oily fish such as herrings, salmon and tuna, butter, margarine, cheese, eggs and liver contain vitamin D. The body can also make vitamin D. Spending half an hour, even in winter, outside with the hands and face exposed to sunlight enables the body to make enough vitamin D for its needs. Elderly people who are housebound and who have a poor diet may develop vitamin D deficiency. People with dark skins are more at risk of developing vitamin D deficiency in the UK. Women who cover their hands and face, such as Muslim women, are at risk of developing vitamin D deficiency.

Vitamin K

Vitamin K is required to enable blood to clot normally. Vitamin K is found in meat and green vegetables. It is also produced by the body in the small intestine. Deficiency is rare.

Special diets

Some older people living in homes require special diets.

Diabetic diet

Older people who suffer from diabetes require a special diet. Normally when we eat, the pancreas produces insulin. Insulin enables us to use the glucose that is produced when food is digested. People who suffer from diabetes either do not produce any insulin or do not produce enough insulin.

There are two different types of diabetes. Type one or insulin dependent diabetes usually occurs when the person is young. It is treated with insulin injections and a diabetic diet. Type two diabetes or non-insulin dependent diabetes, is also known as maturity onset diabetes. The pancreas fails to produce enough insulin for the person's needs. This form of diabetes is less severe than type one diabetes and can sometimes be treated with diet alone. Many people who suffer from type two diabetes are overweight and losing weight helps to control the disease. Some older people are given tablets. These tablets make the pancreas work harder to produce insulin and a combination of tablets and a diabetic diet is used to control diabetes.

Diabetes becomes more common as people age. Research has shown that by the age of 85 one tenth of all older people suffer from diabetes. Some people are more at risk of diabetes than others. Research shows that Asian people are more likely to become diabetic than other races. The reasons for this are not known.

The aim of a diabetic diet is to provide a diet high in fibre and low in fat and sugar. Fresh vegetables and fruit are recommended. The diabetic person can eat starchy foods such as potatoes, but baked potatoes are preferable to chips as they contain more fibre and less fat. The diabetic person should avoid sugar and sweet foods. Diabetics can eat sugar-free puddings. Many desserts are now available that use artificial sweeteners instead of sugar and these are suitable for diabetics. Special biscuits, sweets, chocolates, marmalade and jam can be bought for diabetics.

Overweight diabetics should avoid eating too many 'diabetic' foods. These are sweetened using a substance called sorbitol, which is just as fattening as sugar. Too much sorbitol can cause diarrhoea; a diabetic person who eats a whole packet of sugar free mints or a packet of diabetic custard creams may suffer from acute diarrhoea. Tea and coffee can be sweetened with artificial sweeteners. An artificial sweetener that looks like sugar can be sprinkled over cereals, used to sweeten custard, and used instead of sugar in cakes.

Reducing diets

Reducing diets are intended to help overweight people lose weight. Being overweight can make an older person unwell, and losing weight can make them feel better. People who have high blood pressure and are overweight may find that their blood pressure improves if they lose weight.

People who suffer from arthritis, especially arthritis of the hips and knees, place an extra strain on joints if they are overweight. Losing weight can help reduce pain and increase movement.

The aim of a reducing diet is to produce a small, steady loss in weight. It is important that the older person has a diet with sufficient vitamins and nutrients. Usually the amount of sugar in the diet is reduced. Sweeteners can be used in tea and coffee and on cereals. Fat can be reduced: the older person can have grilled bacon instead of fried, a poached egg instead of a fried egg. Occasional treats such as cake or a small bar of chocolate should be allowed, otherwise the person who is on a reducing diet may decide to give up. If the older person is overweight and does not wish to lose weight, staff working in the home must respect the person's wishes.

Vegetarians

Vegetarians do not eat meat. Some vegetarians eat fish, eggs and dairy products whilst others do not eat any animal products. People who do not eat any animal products are known as vegans. It is important to ensure that people who are vegetarian are offered a healthy vegetarian diet. Details on obtaining information on vegetarian diets appear in the further information section at the end of the chapter.

High fibre diets

High fibre diets help prevent constipation. Further details on the reasons why older people are at risk of developing constipation are given in Chapter 13. A diet rich in fibre can enable older people to have normal bowel actions and avoid relying on laxatives.

There are two different types of fibre: soluble and non-soluble. It is recommended that a high fibre diet should contain a mixture of both types. This means that the diet should contain fruit and vegetables and fibre found in cereals such as porridge, Weetabix, All-bran, wholemeal bread, digestive biscuits and wholemeal flour.

A high fibre diet can be tasty and varied but should be introduced gradually so that the person's body can become used to it. All people are different and the amount of fibre people require varies. One person may find that the diet provides too much fibre and causes diarrhoea, whilst another might require extra fibre perhaps by having an extra portion of fruit, a dish of prunes or a slice of date loaf.

High calorie diet

High calorie diets are required when the older person is thin and undernourished or has increased dietary needs, perhaps because he is more active than other patients, is recovering from a recent operation or has a pressure sore or leg ulcer. The aim is to provide enough calories to meet the patient's needs. Putting too much food on the plate can be off-putting so offer snacks, encourage family and friends to bring in foods that the person is especially fond of, and give dietary supplements if they have been supplied by the doctor.

Puréed diets

Some older people who are very frail or who have difficulty in chewing, perhaps because of a stroke, may require a puréed diet. The aim is to give, as far as possible, a normal diet that has been puréed. Meat and vegetables should not be mixed together and puréed as this is unappetising and the person cannot choose which part of the meal to eat.

Food should be puréed separately. It may be served in a dish with partitions so that the different foods do not blend into each other. Thickening agents are available and the puréed food can be thickened. Moulds can be used to shape puréed food. Puréed thickened lamb can be moulded into a lamb chop mould. Using thickening agents and moulds helps make a puréed diet look more attractive. Sometimes the person receiving a puréed diet may also require dietary supplements.

Meeting the dietary needs of people from different cultures

Some older people come from different backgrounds to those of the majority of people living in homes. People who come from different cultures or who practise different religions may require a different diet. The aim of care in homes is to provide a similar type of life to that which the person would lead living at home. Research shows that although there are a significant number of people from different cultures living in the UK, few people from ethnic minorities enter homes. The reasons for this are not known but there are several theories.

Many people come to the UK from other countries when they are young. In the 1950s, many people came to the UK from the West Indies. They were recruited by London Transport to work on the railways, tubes and buses. Since then, many younger people have entered the UK from other countries. People who came to the UK in the 1950s are only just becoming old and may require care in homes.

Another theory is that already many people from other cultures require care in homes but because homes do not provide special services to meet their needs, they are reluctant to enter homes. It is important that all older people living in homes have their needs met and there cultures respected. People from different cultures have different dietary needs.

Jewish

Jewish people eat a special diet that is called a kosher diet. Those who follow this diet strictly have separate areas within the kitchen for preparing meat and milk dishes. Milk and meat are not eaten together and separate crockery is used for meat and milk dishes. Even people of the Jewish faith who do not have a strict kosher diet normally avoid having meat and milk at the same meal. The person may have cereal with milk for breakfast but would not eat a beef sausage at this meal. Jewish people do not normally eat pork or shellfish. There is a special nursing home in London for Jewish people and a strict kosher diet is available in the home. If a care assistant is caring for a person of the Jewish faith, she should find out what the person prefers to eat and drink.

Muslims

Muslims do not eat pork and normally avoid alcohol. Strict Muslims eat meat that has been killed in a special way, known as halal meat. This can be obtained from halal butchers and is cooked normally. If halal meat is not available, strict Muslims may prefer to avoid eating meat.

Hindus

Hindus do not eat beef. Some people of the Hindu faith are vegetarian and do not eat any animal products.

Dietary supplements

Older people who are unable to eat enough food to meet their requirements are often offered dietary supplements. There is an enormous range of dietary supplements available. These include drinks that look and taste like squash but are high in calories, vitamins and minerals. Other drinks are like milk shakes and come in a range of flavours; these too are full of vitamins, minerals and calories. Special puddings are available, and special high protein snacks such as biscuits may be given.

If the older person appears to be losing weight or is not eating very much, professional advice should be sought. In nursing homes, care assistants will be working under the supervision of registered nurses who will take appropriate action. In residential homes, care assistants should ask the doctor to contact the dietician, who will visit the patient. The dietician will normally bring a range of dietary supplements. The older person can taste these supplements and the dietician will normally contact the patient's doctor and ask for them to be prescribed. Dietary supplements are available on prescription to individuals who have difficulty in swallowing or who suffer from certain conditions.

Why some older people have difficulty eating

Chewing

Chewing can be difficult for some older people. Those who have lost their dentures or who have poorly fitting dentures will have difficulty. People who have suffered from strokes sometimes have difficulty in chewing because one side of the face is paralysed. Confused people, especially those in the advanced stages of dementia, may not be aware that they are supposed to chew food and may leave the food sitting in the mouth unchewed.

Swallowing

Swallowing can be difficult. People who suffer from motor neurone disease, multiple sclerosis, Parkinson's disease or who have suffered from strokes may have difficulty in swallowing. You should encourage people with swallowing difficulties to take small mouthfuls, chew thoroughly and wash food down well with water. The person who has difficulty in swallowing should sit up straight in the chair, as slouching makes the problem worse.

Cutlery

Cutlery can be difficult for some older people to use. The person who has lost the use of one hand may find it very difficult to cut up food and eat one-handed. Special cutlery is available to help people who can only use one hand. People who have severe arthritis in the hands can find it difficult to grip ordinary cutlery, and special cutlery is available for them.

Some people find that the plate slips. Non-slip mats placed under the plate prevent this. If a person is eating one-handed, the food can easily slip off the plate. Using a plate guard that clips onto the plate prevents this. Aids to help older people to eat can be purchased from medical supplies companies or they can be supplied by the occupational therapist for the individual's use. The patient's doctor can ask the occupational therapist to visit to provide suitable aids. Aids can enable even the most disabled people to eat independently. Figure 6.2 shows such an aid.

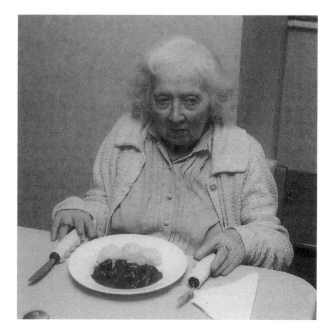

Fig. 6.2   Resident with arthritic hands using special cutlery.

Poor eyesight
Poor eyesight can prevent people from seeing the food on the plate. Using dark coloured plates to provide a contrast enables the older person to see the food more easily.

Confusion
Most residents who are confused have dementia. People who have dementia have great difficulty processing information. Too much bustle and too many things happening at once cause great distress. Some confused people can find it difficult to settle down to eat a meal. Creating a relaxed, calm atmosphere helps confused people to settle and enjoy their meal. Turning off the television, playing music and avoiding bustling about help to create a relaxing mealtime. Research carried out in American nursing homes found that when lighting was subdued and gentle music was played residents ate more. Residents became unsettled

when country and western music was played but relaxed and ate well when classical music or nature sounds were played.

In some cases confused residents benefit from eating in a small dining room where bustle can be reduced to a minimum.

Serving food and making mealtimes a pleasure

Mealtimes should be pleasant occasions and should give the older person the opportunity not only to enjoy a meal but also to chat with others and to relax over the meal. It is important that staff make an effort to make eating a pleasant experience. In many nursing homes, breakfast is served in the patient's room. The older person should be made comfortable for breakfast and helped to sit up in bed or to sit out in a chair if she requires help. Food should be presented attractively and served hot; lukewarm tea and cold porridge do not encourage people to eat.

Many homes encourage older people to eat lunch in the dining room so that they can chat with others. Tables should be set out with tablecloths, napkins, cutlery, drinks, salt, pepper and sauces. Older people who are able to help lay tables should be encouraged to do so. Playing music quietly in the background helps create a relaxing atmosphere and encourages people to relax and enjoy their meal. People who require help with eating can be helped by care assistants. You should sit down with the individual who requires help, as this makes the person feel more relaxed and less hurried.

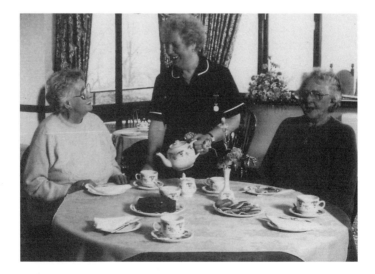

Fig. 6.3 Residents enjoying their tea.

Preparing food and drink

Care assistants in most homes are rarely required to cook main meals. Many care assistants may prepare snacks to tempt people with poor appetites to eat. Occasionally you may be required to help in the kitchen. Most homes now employ a cook or chef who is responsible for meals.

When preparing food and drink it is important to remember that we eat with our eyes. Presentation is very important. All the presentation in the world is wasted if the food provided is not what the person wants so it is important to find out what the person wishes to eat.

Enabling people to choose

Information about enabling people to choose drinks is given earlier in the chapter. Choosing what to eat is something we take for granted. Yet many people living in homes have difficulty choosing food. There are many reasons for this.

Poor vision can make it difficult for people to read the menu. People who have had strokes may no longer be able to read. People who do not read English will be unable to choose from a menu written in English.

Some older people are expected to tick boxes on a menu to indicate their choices. People who are no longer able to write cannot complete such menus.

Some older people have poor memories. The person may choose a dish for the next day but forget by morning. There are many ways you can enable people to choose what they would like to eat. Some suggestions include:

- Produce the menu in large print; many older people with visual problems can read 20 point bold with ease
- Use pictures to illustrate the menu – if offering fish and chips cut out a picture of fish and chips and stick it next to the writing; people who are unable to read can see the pictures of the dishes and point
- Allow people to choose their next meal as late as possible; in the home where I worked residents were able to choose lunch up to 11AM that morning
- Read the menu to people with visual problems
- Note people's likes and dislikes in the care plan

Summary

Eating and drinking are essential if the individual is to remain in good health. Some older people living in homes require help to eat and drink; others, especially those with special dietary needs, may require advice on what foods they should eat. Care assistants should be aware of the older person's fluid and food preferences. You should aim to provide, wherever possible, food and drink that the older person prefers. The food available should be similar to that which the older person would choose to eat at home. Care assistants should offer to assist older people who require help and should be careful to ensure that the older person maintains dignity at all times.

Portfolio preparation

Your assessor must have evidence that you can meet the performance criteria for these units. Before beginning these units discuss assessment strategies with your assessor. Most of the evidence for these units can be gained by direct observation of your work. You may be asked to provide the following types of evidence.

■ Products. This might include a copy of a fluid balance chart that you have completed. Remember to delete the resident's name to preserve confidentiality.
■ Witness testimony. This is a statement from a senior member of staff and might be a statement detailing how you have met certain performance criteria.
■ Written work. You might be asked to prepare a piece of work about how you encourage a resident to eat a balanced diet, or you might be asked to write a case history about a resident with special dietary needs and how those are met.

Your assessor will also use other methods to help you gain evidence for this unit. These may include:

■ Verbal questioning
■ Written questions

Simulations can be used to increase your awareness of how it feels to be fed. Some assessors ask students to feed each other and then discuss their feelings. Often students report that they are fed too quickly, not told what they are having or that the spoon is overloaded. This type of simulation improves care.

Simulations can also be used to assess your ability to meet performance criteria.

Further information

The British Diabetic Association (BDA)
10 Queen Anne Street
London W1M 0BD
Tel. 020 7323 1531
Information on all aspects of diabetes and diabetic diets is available. They produce a range of leaflets, books and videos and will send a catalogue on request.

Vegetarian Society
Park Dale
Durham Road
Altringham
Cheshire WA14 4QG
Tel. 0161 925 2000
Information on vegetarian diets is available. They produce a useful leaflet, *Healthy Nutrition in Later Life*, which contains guidance and recipes and is available free if an SAE is sent.

Kellogg's Education Pack
Freepost
Horndean
Waterlooville
Hants PO8 9BR
Information on high fibre diets is available. They produce a patient education pack and a selection of recipes.

Unigreg Ltd
Enterprise House
181–189 Garth Road
Morden
Surrey SM4 4LL
Tel. 020 8330 1421
Nutritional helpline 0800 373 698, 9AM–5.30PM Monday to Friday.
E-mail: admin@unigreg.co.uk
Unigreg produce vitamins. The company provides a nutritional helpline and a range of educational materials including a booklet, *Understanding Nutrition*.

Further reading

Nursing Times (1998) *Nutrition in Practice*. This binder contains ten articles on nutrition including one on nutrition and the elderly. You may find it in your college library.

Sandy, D. (1997) *Food in Care*. MacMillan Caring Series. This book provides detailed advice on nutrition. You may find it in your college library.

Chapter 7

Supporting Older People and their Families

Introduction

This chapter covers the option group A units W2, W2.1, W2.2, W2.3, and W2.4 – 'contribute to the ongoing support of clients and others significant to their needs'. This unit applies to people living in their own homes receiving care, people living in nursing and residential homes and people receiving treatment in hospital. This chapter will focus on people living in nursing and residential homes. The option group B units W8, W8.1 and W8.2 – 'enable individuals to maintain contacts in potentially isolating situation' – is covered in the first section of this chapter. The option group B units Z13, Z13.1 and Z13.2 – 'enable clients to participate in recreation and leisure activities' – are covered in the second section of this chapter.

This chapter gives information on:

- Living at home
- Life in a home
- Enabling older people to retain their identities and interests
- How families feel about homes
- How staff view families
- Helping, supporting and welcoming families and friends
- Enabling older people to see visitors in private
- The benefits of activities and interests
- Activities and interests

Life at home

Most older people live independent lives and do not require care. The people who enter homes are the most frail and ill of their generation. It is easy for us to lose sight of this when working in homes and to assume that all 85-year-old women have difficulty in caring for themselves. It is also easy for us to forget that the person who has come to the home may until recently have been living a full and independent life in his or her own home.

Doris Smith is a widow who has lived alone for five years. She decides what time to get up, what to eat for breakfast, when to wash, what to eat for lunch, what to do during the day. She decides to listen to the radio or read a book or watch television.

Entering a home

Suddenly Mrs Smith's life is shattered. She suffers a stroke. A few weeks after the stroke she is visited by her family and the care manager who inform her that she will not be able to manage at home any more. A home is suggested. Mrs Smith is informed that she needs long-term care. This will mean having to give up her home, clear the house full of memories and the possessions of a lifetime and enter a home.

Suddenly Mrs Smith, who has always valued her independence and declined offers to move in with her daughter, is no longer in control. The home she enters is clean and tidy but she cannot bring her own furniture. The home has a routine and because Mrs Smith has difficulty in communicating, the staff do not realise that she is alert. Mrs Smith is 'got up' when it is convenient for the staff. Breakfast is at 8AM and no one asks Mrs Smith if she would prefer to eat earlier or later. Mrs Smith has some difficulty in swallowing because of the stroke, so she has porridge, tea, white bread, butter and marmalade for breakfast. Mrs Smith would love a lightly poached egg on brown bread and a cup of black coffee.

Mrs Smith is bathed twice a week on Sundays and Wednesdays and is bedbathed on all other days. She prefers to shower each day. Mrs Smith's daughter has brought her clothes in from home. Her wardrobe, like every other woman's, contains clothes she rarely wears because she has 'gone off' them. Now no one asks her what she likes to wear and she is often dressed in that red dress she kept meaning to throw out. Mrs Smith is not able to make any real choices about her life. She is dependent on the staff at the home to help her. If she is sat next to someone with whom she has little in common she cannot go and sit elsewhere.

Enabling older people to retain their identities

Mrs Smith's fictional experience may seem far-fetched but it shows how easy it is for people to lose their identities just because they are old and sick. Mrs Smith has entered the home at her lowest ebb. Staff who realise this, get to know her as a person and take time to discover her needs and wishes will make a real difference to her quality of life.

Mrs Smith would benefit from a full assessment by a speech and language therapist who could advise staff of the best ways to help Mrs Smith communicate. In the meantime, staff could take time to find out Mrs Smith's wishes – further details are given in Chapter 2. Mrs Smith's daughter could help and advise staff. She would be able to tell them that Mrs Smith prefers black coffee, has never liked that red dress and would feel much better if her hair was cut and permed in her normal style. Mrs Smith and the staff could begin to form a relationship and work together to help her regain as much independence as possible.

Seeing someone like Mrs Smith enter a home feeling that it is the end of the world, and having the opportunity to work with her and see her improve mentally and physically, is so rewarding. It is, after all, the reason we all decided to work with older people.

Living life to the full

Often when we ask people what they do for a living, we learn a lot about them. In some homes, staff do not know very much about the older person's life. Is Mr Robinson a retired schoolteacher or a mechanic? If we are to help older people to retain their identities when living in homes, we need to know who they are. What is the older person's background? What interests has that person followed throughout life? In some homes staff keep a book and enter details of the person's life, interests, likes and dislikes. This can help all staff not only to see the whole person but also to give care that the person wants.

Mrs Anderson for example is a retired music teacher. Her eyesight is fading but she enjoys listening to music on the radio or television. Julie Carson, a care assistant at the home, checks the radio and television programmes each week and marks any which she feels will interest Mrs Anderson. Julie then discusses these with Mrs Anderson and when Mrs Anderson has decided which she would like to hear, a note of them is made. Staff help Mrs Anderson to sit comfortably in her room and make sure that the radio or television is on the right channel for her to enjoy her concert.

Mrs Anderson dislikes Brussels sprouts, gravy, semolina, and too much custard on her puddings. A note of her likes and dislikes has been made. Mrs Anderson has been able to retain her identity and is treated as an individual. This is good for her morale. It makes her feel cared for and valued. We all feel so much better when we are treated as individuals, and older people are no different to you and I.

Homes – the family's view

Many older people are cared for at home, before they enter homes. Others are living independent lives before an illness such as a stroke leads to hospital admission. The average older person living in a home is 85 years old. The older person's children are often retired and in their sixties and seventies. Many families feel that they have 'failed' when an older person is admitted to a home. Some families feel guilty that they could not care for the older person at home. Most older people who are admitted to homes require high levels of care and in most cases it would be impossible to provide this level of care at home, especially on a long-term basis. Some older people do not realise how much care they require and constantly ask their families to take them home. Many relatives are anxious about the care the home will offer; they worry about their loved one receiving the care and attention required.

Some relatives have struggled alone and without help, or the specialist equipment that the home has, until they reach the end of their tether. The older person is admitted to the home and if care appears good, the relative can feel inadequate, perhaps thinking, 'Look how well the staff cope, yet I couldn't even look after my own mother'. In other cases the relative may be very critical of the care in the home and may think, 'What have I done putting her into a home?'

People who suffer from dementia gradually lose the ability to remember. In the end stages of the disease the older person no longer recognises herself in the mirror and is often unable to recognise her family. A daughter who visits her mother in the home to find that her mother no longer recognises her can become terribly upset by this. Sometimes relatives find visiting very painful. If staff do not recognise this distress, they may label the relative uncaring. The relative can grow to dread not only seeing her mother but also facing the staff.

Case history

Mrs Phyllis Banes was admitted to St Michael's because of severe dementia. Her daughter Lucy seldom visited and barely spoke to staff. Ellen Gray, the matron of the nursing home, noticed that Lucy sat in the car around 20 minutes before rushing in white and tight-lipped to visit her mother. When Ellen mentioned this to Lucy she broke down in tears and explained that she found visiting her mother so painful that she had to steel herself to come in. 'Mum doesn't know who I am. When I come, she says you can't be my Lucy, she's just a little girl. Go away.' The woman whom staff thought was uninterested desperately needed help and support to enable her to come to terms with her mother's illness.

The staff view

Staff sometimes feel that they cannot win with relatives. If the older person looks and feels well the relative feels guilty; if the older person appears unsettled and asks to go home the staff are not providing good care. Some relatives visit daily and appear to ask for information about every little detail of the patient's day. Others visit rarely and appear to take no interest in the patient.

Helping and supporting families

The older person's family want the best possible care for their loved one. Staff want to care for older people and to give the best possible care. Families and staff who work together as a team can make sure that the care the older person receives is of the best possible standard. It is important to make time to get to know the older person's family and build up a good relationship. When the older person enters a home, the family may be anxious and upset. The care assistant who understands the reasons why families feel this way will be able to build a relationship with the family.

Homes are much busier than before. Once the average older person entering a nursing home lived there for 22 months. The average older person entering a residential home lived there for 34 months. Now people are being admitted to nursing and residential homes later than they once were. Increasingly nursing and residential homes are providing respite care to give families who are caring for a relative a break. Now the average stay in nursing homes is around 13 weeks, in residential homes it is around 28 weeks. This means that staff are busier, there are more admissions and there is less time to spend building up a relationship with families. Despite these pressures, it is important that you spend time getting to know the resident's family.

Families often feel that they can no longer have any say in the older person's life because they have 'handed over' to the staff at the home. Relatives have known their loved one for a lifetime and know much more about the person than the staff do. If you ask relatives for their help and advice, they will feel that they can continue to have some influence over the older person's life. The care assistant who chats to a relative might say, 'Yes, it is lovely today. I was going to ask if Mrs Harrison would like me to take her to the shops in her wheelchair later. Do you think she'd like that?' The skilled care assistant can discuss how Mrs Harrison enjoys her trips to the shops when her daughter next visits. Within a few weeks, Mrs Harrison's daughter may be taking her mother to the shops when she visits.

Relatives who cared for their loved one at home may feel

failures when the older person enters a home. The care assistant who asks the relative for advice immediately builds a bond with the relative; for example, you might ask:

'I noticed that Mrs Kay's skin is very dry. Has she had this problem before'.

'Yes. I tried lots of creams but they weren't much good. In the end, the doctor prescribed a cream that worked well. Would you like me to get the name of it for you? I think I've got it in my bag.'

When a relative has cared for a loved one at home the older person often becomes the centre of the relative's life. The relative may have dropped outside interests and lost touch with friends because all free time was devoted to caring. In such circumstances, relatives may be relieved that the loved one is happy and well cared for in a home.

The relative may, however, feel guilty and may ask you to assure her that she has done the right thing:

'You must think I'm wicked.'

'I do feel terrible about Mum being here, but she seems very happy.'

The care assistant might reply, 'She is happy but she does need a lot of care. It's easier for us here. We go home at night and the night staff take over. You did really well to care for her so well at home for such a long time.'

The care assistant is letting the relative know that the staff are not judging her and that they realise that caring for a loved one at home is not always possible.

In most areas the local council appoints a carers support co-ordinator. There are usually a number of local carers support groups, who meet regularly. Some members are carers and others are people who have a family member in a home. Relatives attending these groups can talk to other people in similar situations. The groups also organise social activities and this gives relatives the opportunity to meet others socially. The carers support co-ordinator can supply details of local groups. If your home does not have a contact number this can be obtained from the Citizen's Advice Bureau or the social services department in your town hall.

Helping families to remain involved

Many relatives are keen to remain involved in caring for their loved one. Some do not offer because they worry about offending staff. Other relatives have seen their loved one change from a healthy independent person to a disabled person. This change can literally happen overnight.

Case history

Mr Charles Webster was widowed some years ago. He remained active and did all his own shopping, cooking, cleaning and ironing. He visited his local pub twice a week and met his friends. One winter's evening he slipped over on the pavement on his way to the pub. He fell heavily and broke his leg. Surgeons at the local hospital operated but unfortunately Mr Webster suffered a heart attack. He was discharged to a home, unable to walk or care for himself.

Mr Webster gradually learnt to walk again and became more independent. He was unable to walk long distances because of his heart condition. His son often visited the home and staff noticed that both father and son ran out of conversation after a few minutes. Both looked awkward. One of the care assistants, Lily McDonald, asked how they normally spent their time together before Mr Webster's illness. She learnt that father and son normally went to the pub and had a chat over a pint. Lily suggested that they go to the pub during visits and offered to fetch a wheelchair so that the son could push his father to the pub. His son was frightened by the suggestion and thought that because his father had been ill he could not go out without a member of staff; it was too dangerous, anything might happen. He agreed to take his father to the pub if a member of staff accompanied them 'just in case'. After a few visits both father and son felt confident to go to the pub unaccompanied – much to the disappointment of staff!

Some relatives are equally worried about having a loved one home to tea. You can help by encouraging relatives and by offering to accompany the family on a trial visit. This can help everyone feel more confident. Relatives can often help and encourage exercises and therapy; for example, if an older person has speech difficulties after a stroke, staff can involve caring relatives in therapy.

Case history

Mrs Winifred Pearson was admitted to a home from hospital following a stroke. She was unable to speak. She was visited by a speech and language therapist who carried out an assessment and worked out a plan of care. Mrs Pearson's family took a day off work and met the speech and language therapist at the home. They worked with the staff at the home to help Mrs Pearson regain her speech.

Visiting

Visiting times

The home is now the older person's home. At home, the older person would welcome friends and relatives. It is important that the home encourages the older person's family and friends to visit, and makes them feel welcome. Hospitals have visiting hours, and restricting visiting to certain hours helps ensure that hospital patients get enough rest and that treatment can be carried out. Hospital visiting hours are now more flexible than before and are normally from 2PM until 8PM. Some hospitals have open visiting policies but others are beginning to re-introduce visiting hours, saying that patients need to rest.

Many homes do not have set visiting hours and welcome people throughout the day. Find out what the policy on visiting hours is in your home. Homes aim to provide care in a setting that is as normal and home-like as possible. At home, people call when they are passing and when they have time. If the home has rigid visiting hours, this can make it difficult for some people to visit and can put others off.

Some home managers fear that if there are no set visiting hours, the home will be over-run with visitors and it will be difficult to care for patients. This is not the case. An open visiting policy encourages people to visit and is probably less disruptive than a rush of visitors at 2PM on Sunday afternoons. Family, friends and neighbours can pop in and do not expect the home to look perfect at all times. If a doctor or therapist has arrived, visitors will leave if required and can return later.

Many older people look forward to visits from old friends of their own age group. If visiting hours start at 2PM and the visitor stays a few hours, he or she may have to travel home in the dark on a winter's evening. The prospect of this can put some older people off visiting and can deprive patients of the company of their dearest friends.

Some relatives work and if visiting ends at 8PM, for example, the relative may have to rush straight from work to the home. The relative may be tired and hungry and may only visit for a short time. Sometimes the relative may decide not to visit. If relatives can visit later in the evening, there is time to go home, eat and relax before the visit. The relative will be encouraged to visit more often and stay longer.

Many older people in homes look forward to visits but too many visitors at once can be tiring; an open visiting policy enables people to spread their visits through the day. The older person has an opportunity to chat at length with each visitor. Some older people go to bed early in the evening because they are bored and have nothing to look forward to. An evening visit brightens the evening and prevents boredom. Proposed national required standards require all homes to have an open visiting policy.

Welcoming visitors

Many visitors travel long distances to visit the home; others have come direct from work. It is normal to offer visitors refreshments when they visit our own homes and offering visitors a cup of tea or coffee makes them feel welcome. At times, the home may be busy and it can be difficult to find time to make tea. Perhaps your home could offer tea and coffee making facilities so that visitors can help themselves in such circumstances.

Privacy during visits

Some older people have difficulty hearing. They may not enjoy a visit if they have to strain to hear above background noise in a lounge. Everyone has the right to privacy during visits. Some people prefer to remain in a communal area, such as a lounge, while others prefer to see their visitors in the privacy of their room. Some older people have difficulty in walking and require assistance to get to and from their rooms. Carers should be sensitive to the needs of visitors and patients and should offer to assist patients to their rooms if they wish to enjoy a visit in private.

Visitors can be encouraged to take the older person out on short trips to the shops, to the local cafe or to the park if they wish. All 'visits' do not have to take place within the home. Check how your home encourages and involves visitors.

Helping residents maintain contact with family and friends

Sometimes friends and family are unable to visit as often as they would like. The individual may have family who live far away. Sometimes a lifelong friend may live nearby but is too infirm to travel. It is important to do everything you can to help the individual maintain contact in these circumstances.

Case history

Mrs Enid Lovelace lived in St Michael's nursing home in London. Her only living relative was her sister Edith. Edith lived in Greenbanks residential home in Eastbourne. The sisters maintained contact by sending each other notelets and postcards. Staff at Greenbanks helped Edith to write the card. Staff at St Michael's read the card to Enid whose sight was failing. Every Sunday at 10AM the sisters would speak on the telephone. On the first Saturday of every month one of the sisters would be driven to visit the other. The staff at both homes worked to enable the sisters to remain in touch.

It can be difficult to enable people who have problems with hearing or sight to remain in touch but where there's a will, there's a way. The solutions are only limited by our imagination.

Case history

Maud Black's young brother, Cyril, who was 92, travelled from Harrogate to Kent several times a year. He also wrote to his sister twice a week. When Cyril lost his sight staff helped Maud tape messages to her brother and to play the messages he sent her.

Summary

Older people living in their own home make decisions about their lives. They are free to pursue their own interests and to welcome family, friends and neighbours into their homes. Staff should aim to enable older people living in homes to live as full a life as possible within the home. Each person is unique and has their own personality and interests; carers should work with older people and their families to help people retain their interests.

Families often worry and feel guilty when a loved one enters a home; they want only the best for their loved one. The relationship that care assistants build up with the older person's friends and family is just as important as the one between staff and residents. Enabling residents to keep in touch with their loved ones helps the older person to preserve identity. Offering a flexible, sensitive and welcoming environment encourages people to drop in and keep in touch. The person living in the home feels that he is not abandoned but still part of the family. This helps the person feel wanted and is good for morale. The person who feels that he is not forgotten will enjoy the best possible quality of life.

Portfolio preparation

Your assessor must have evidence that you can meet the performance criteria for these units. Before beginning these units discuss assessment strategies with your assessor. Most of the evidence for these units can be gained by direct observation of your work. You may be asked to provide the following types of evidence.

- Products. This might include a copy of a letter that you have written for a resident. You must obtain the person's permission to copy the letter, postcard or note. Remember to delete the name and address to preserve confidentiality.
- Witness testimony. This is a statement from a senior member of staff, a relative or a resident. This might be a statement detailing how you have met certain performance criteria. Remember to ask a senior member of staff before asking a

relative or resident for a witness testimony. This will seldom be a problem but it is a matter of courtesy. The statement could be recorded on a tape if the person is unable to write. It could be dictated, written down, and witnessed by a senior member of staff.

■ Written work. You might be asked to prepare a piece of work about how you enable residents to maintain contact with friends and family. You might be asked to write a case history about a resident whom you have helped maintain links with family. You might be asked to write a case history about how you have helped a particular relative or friend to keep in touch.

Your assessor will also use other methods to help you gain evidence for this unit. These may include:

■ Verbal questioning
■ Written questions

Role-play can be used to increase your awareness of how it feels to be a relative or friend of an older person. Often students report that they see the home and the staff with new eyes when asked to assume the role of a relative. Role-play can also be used to assess your ability to meet performance criteria.

Benefit of activities and interests

This section covers the option group B units Z13, Z13.1, and Z13.2 – 'enable clients to participate in recreation and leisure activities'.

Homes are for living in and activities and interests make life worthwhile and interesting for many people. Activities have been shown to improve concentration and reduce boredom. Taking part in activities helps people to live full lives and this improves physical and mental wellbeing.

In the early 1980s, many older people requiring long-term care were cared for in NHS units. These units were usually in geriatric hospitals built many years before. Older people were nursed in wards. There was little privacy and they were dressed in clothes supplied by the hospital laundry rather than in their own clothes. In many hospitals, older people were not treated as individuals and there were few opportunities for them to pursue their interests.

It was thought that older people would enjoy a better quality of life if they were cared for in nursing homes. Four experimental nursing homes were set up and people were asked if they wished to move from the hospital to the nursing home. The homes aimed to provide care in an environment that was more like the older person's home than a hospital. Individuals had their own rooms, wore their own clothes and were encouraged to take part in activities and pursue their own interests.

The results were dramatic; people who had lived in hospital for years began to take an interest in life again and their physical and mental health improved. Activities encourage older people to move around, to sit up, to concentrate and to take an interest in life. People who are more alert and involved are less likely to spend half the day dozing in the chair and will normally sleep well at night without sleeping tablets.

Encouraging individual activities and interests

People come from many different backgrounds and they have different skills, interests, experiences, and personalities. Older people who live in homes differ in their interests just as much as any other group of people. The activities offered in the home should take account of the different interests and personalities of the people living there. Some people are naturally chatty and outgoing and love company. Some patients rush to get ready and get to the lounge for coffee and a chat. Others are quieter and prefer to spend their days quietly away from the bustle and activity of others. In some homes, patients are placed under some pressure by well-meaning staff to join in activities that have been organised.

If a person does not wish to take part in an activity you should ask why; some people long to join in but lack confidence. You can help, support and encourage patients who lack confidence, to take part in activities. Some older people are embarrassed by their disabilities or worry that because of illness it will be difficult to participate. You can help by encouraging and offering practical help in such situations. Activities in the home should be organised to take account of disabilities and to enable individuals to participate. Some older people prefer their own company or that of their family and friends who visit. If the individual prefers not to take part in activities, you should respect their wishes.

Organising activities

Many larger homes employ an activities organiser. This person works with staff and residents to organise and co-ordinate activities within the home. Many people, when they think of activities, imagine a large group of people all doing the same thing. Well-organised activity programmes involve working with small groups of people and with individuals as well as large groups. At some homes a number of people come to the home for a few sessions each week. Activity sessions from different people offer a variety of activities.

In smaller homes, staff are required to work with patients to organise activities. In this situation staff have to ensure that activities are not squeezed out by the other work in the home. Homes are busy places and there is always something to do. Activities are important and helping patients to pursue their interests and activities is a very important part of working in homes. Ask any older person what mattered most to them: the person who tidied the lockers, or the one who found time to help residents begin a game of Scrabble.

Types of activities

If you are involved in activity programmes aim to offer as wide a range of activities as possible. It is easy for people to become bored if only a limited range of activities is offered.

Games
Many older people enjoy games. Some older people have poor eyesight even with spectacles. Playing cards that are twice the normal size can be seen by people with poor eyesight. A large print version of Scrabble is available. People with poor eyesight can see this more easily and people suffering from diseases such as motor neurone disease, multiple sclerosis and arthritis will find them easier to handle.

Large easy-to-handle draughts are also available. Bingo is popular in many homes. Large print bingo cards are available. Many homes have radios or music centres, which have microphones. The microphone can be used to call numbers so that people who do not have perfect hearing can join in.

Music
Many people enjoy music. It is easy to build up a record collection for the home. A notice on the home's notice board and a letter to the local newspaper asking for records usually works well. If you ask what type of music people prefer you will normally find this varies from classical to popular music of the 1920s, 1930s and 1940s. In some homes, popular music is played during the morning and classical in the evening.

Most local hospitals have hospital radio stations, and many of these also offer a tape service. A member of the radio team visits the home and speaks to a group of residents asking what type of music they prefer. The music is then taped and sent to the home. Tapes are usually exchanged twice weekly. Individuals can also have a personal selection of music taped and sent to them regularly. This can be listened to in private or enjoyed with others.

Singsongs can also be popular. Tapes or records of favourite songs from musicals such as *South Pacific* can be bought. It is often possible to buy large print songbooks that help people join in. If songbooks are not available, the words can be typed out and printed in large print by someone with access to a computer. You can help by encouraging residents to join in and by joining in yourself.

Many homes have pianos that are seldom used because no one can play. Often a notice saying 'Volunteer wanted to play the piano for one hour a week' will bring offers flooding in. An advertisement in a newsagent's window costs very little. Many local supermarkets offer a free notice board service, so it may be worth advertising. The local secondary school may have pupils who would enjoy playing.

Concerts

Concerts can be formal and involve the use of professional entertainers, but this can be expensive and your home may not be able to afford many such concerts. Local choirs, operatic societies and other groups may be willing to perform in the home. Details of local groups can be obtained from your local library or Citizens Advice Bureau.

Arts and crafts

Painting and drawing are relaxing activities. Many people who are no longer able to take part in more active pursuits enjoy creating drawings, pictures, prints and collages. Some older people are talented artists and create impressive paintings, whilst others enjoy making birthday cards, Christmas cards and prints. Paper, pencils, pens, felt-tip pens and poster paints are inexpensive and give hours of pleasure (Fig. 7.1). When people have worked hard to produce work it can be admired and displayed in the person's room or in the lounge, dining room and hall.

Many women enjoy knitting. Some, though able to knit beautifully, find that it is difficult to read a pattern because the print is too small. They could use a magnifier, or large print knitting patterns are available from Carter & Parker Ltd, Gordon Mills, Guiseley, Leeds LS20 9PD. People who have poor eyesight but are still able to knit may have difficulty sewing up garments. Often another resident who enjoys sewing may be able to help finish off garments. Both may enjoy working together.

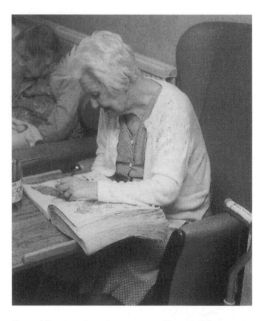

Fig. 7.1   A resident colouring – not all activities are group activities.

Pets

Most people who enter homes lived alone before entering the home. This may be because they never married or because they were widowed. Many people who live alone enjoy the companionship of pets. People who live alone and who have pets enjoy better health than those without pets. Stroking a cat or patting a dog has been shown to reduce blood pressure and help people to relax.

Some homes have a policy of allowing the older person with a pet to bring the pet to live at the home wherever possible. This is not always possible, however, as some breeds of dog require a lot of exercise and the older person who enters a home will rarely be able to take a dog for long walks. Many older people recognise these difficulties and ask a friend or relative to care for their dog when they enter a home. Most homes now encourage family and friends to bring the older person's dog to visit. Many other residents also enjoy such visits. Cats require less looking after and in some homes the older person may bring her cat to stay.

Case history

Grace Andrews was admitted to a nursing home after suffering from a severe stroke. She recovered well from the stroke and regained speech and mobility but remained quiet and withdrawn. Staff at the home discovered that when Mrs Andrews was in hospital her cat had been run over and killed. Mrs Andrews missed the companionship dreadfully. The local Cats Protection League visited and Mrs Andrews 'adopted' a cat. Having the companionship of a cat made Mrs Andrews feel that life was worth living again (Fig. 7.2).

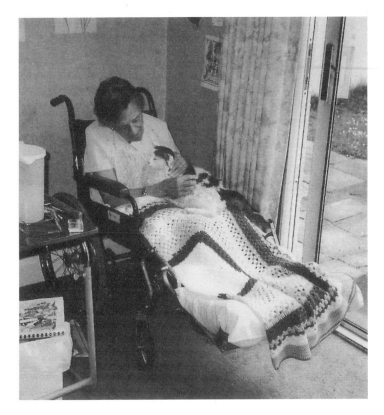

Fig. 7.2   Grace and her cat.

Some people have budgies as pets and most homes allow people to bring these with them when they enter the home.

Sport

Recently researchers asked older men living in nursing and residential homes what would improve their quality of life most within the home. A huge majority said they would like satellite television so that they could watch the sport. Many older people enjoy watching sport. Football, boxing, tennis, horse racing and cricket are often shown on television, although increasingly satellite television has more coverage of major sporting events. If an individual enjoys watching, carers can help by checking the times of particular events and helping the person to enjoy them uninterrupted. The person who enjoys tennis should have chiropody treatment planned so that it will not coincide with matches at Wimbledon.

Many people enjoy watching sports events out of doors. If Mr Walters played rugby as a younger man, he may enjoy watching a local rugby team. The team can be contacted and arrangements made for him to watch local matches. Many sports teams are extremely helpful and will help transport sports enthusiasts to their games and involve them in the social activities of the team. Sitting under a tree watching a cricket match or sitting in a pub watching the darts team play is a world away from how most people view homes. You can, with a little imagination and planning, help older people live life to the full within homes.

Exercise sessions
Exercise is not only for the young and fit. People of all ages can benefit from exercise; even frail and disabled people can take part. EXTEND (Exercise Training For the Elderly) is a charity which specialises in working with older people. Using music and a series of exercises that exercise different parts of the body, EXTEND aims to make people living in homes feel as well as possible.

Reading
Homes obtain books from the mobile library service, which is run by the local council. Councils deliver a selection of books to homes and hospitals, and these are exchanged every few months. The library service ask the home which types of books are required. Most older people find it easier to read large print and there is now a large selection of large print books available. If an older person is an avid reader, the library service can deliver a book (or two) to the individual. The library asks the person to fill in a form (usually large print) asking them their reading preferences and delivers and collects books on request. Some older people may prefer to go to the library and select their own books. You can escort and help individuals who wish to do this. You can also suggest that family and friends take the individual to the local library to select books.

Books for the blind and partially sighted
People who have very poor vision can be registered blind. The patient's doctor fills in a form and the person is registered with the local council. People who are registered blind or partially sighted are issued with special library tickets that enable them to take out tapes or books free of charge. There are two sizes of book tape. The Talking Book cassette recorders take larger cassettes. Talking Book cassettes are posted to registered blind people from a central library run by the council. The book cassettes available in local libraries fit into normal cassette players. Older people with poor

vision can find it difficult to use standard cassette players. Some older people with poor vision find that cassette players designed for toddlers are easy to use. These are inexpensive and easy to obtain. There are four large bright differently coloured buttons each with a separate function.

Television and films
Many older people enjoy watching television. It is important though that television is not seen as the only activity. In some homes, the television is on all day and no one is listening. Try to find out which television programmes individual residents like and let them know when these are on. Many people like watching films, especially old films. Many classic films are inexpensive and can be obtained easily. If the home has a video recorder films can be taped and film shows organised in the evening. This can be made into an event, with drinks and popcorn available.

Gardening
Gardening is a popular pastime for people of all ages. People living in homes will have differing abilities. Some suggestions to enable people who enjoy gardening to continue their interest are:

- Caring for a raised bed or a tub of plants in the garden.
- Planting indoor bulbs. Bulbs can be planted all year round. Bulbs can be planted in bowls and containers to brighten up the person's bedroom or other parts of the home.
- Planting seeds. Usually large seeds such as nasturtium are easier to handle. Choose plants that germinate easily. There's nothing worse than watching and waiting for plants that fail to sprout. Plants can be transferred into pots, bowls, tubs or the garden.
- Taking cuttings from plants. Residents can give the new plants to family and friends as gifts.

Outings
Many people enjoy going out and often people in homes enjoy outings. Some homes successfully organise regular outings, while others are less successful. If you are involved in planning an outing:

- Do not think that the aim is to take every resident. It is better to organise several smaller outings as older people, like all of us, have differing interests.
- Find out what residents require.
- Plan the outing. Visit the place beforehand to make sure it is suitable.
- Involve families and friends. Ask for help and support.
- Remember things rarely go exactly to plan, so be flexible.

Individual activities

Some people who come to live in homes have managed their own leisure activities for years. In such circumstances, your role should be to support the person and offer help if required. If the person is a member of the local bridge club then your role may be to welcome visitors and offer them refreshments.

Portfolio preparation

Your assessor must have evidence that you can meet the performance criteria for these units. Before beginning these units discuss assessment strategies with your assessor. Most of the evidence for these units can be gained by direct observation of your work. You may be asked to provide the following types of evidence:

- Products. This might include details of an activity you have organised. One NVQ level 2 student organised a Christmas pantomime and submitted a video recording of the pantomime in her evidence. Another organised a trip to the seaside and submitted photographs of residents enjoying the trip.
- Witness testimony. This is a statement from a senior member of staff, a relative or a resident. This might be a statement detailing how you have met certain performance criteria. Remember to ask a senior member of staff before asking a relative or resident for a witness testimony. This will seldom be a problem but it is a matter of courtesy. The statement could be recorded on a tape if the person is unable to write. It could be dictated, written down and witnessed by a senior member of staff.
- Written work. You might be asked to prepare a piece of work about how you enable residents to maintain their interests or develop new ones in the home. You might be asked to write a case history about a resident whom you have helped maintain links with family. You might be asked to write a case history about how you have helped a particular relative or friend keep in touch.

Your assessor will also use other methods to help you gain evidence for this unit. These may include:

- Verbal questioning
- Written questions

Role-play can be used to increase your awareness of how it feels to be a relative or friend of an older person. Often students report that they see the home and the staff with new eyes when asked to assume the role of a relative.

Role-play can also be used to assess your ability to meet performance criteria.

Further information

The Relatives and Residents Association
5 Tavistock Place
London WC1H 9SN
Tel. 020 7916 6055
The Relatives and Residents Association is an organisation for relatives and friends of people who live in nursing and residential homes and NHS continuing care units. The Relatives and Residents Association runs an information and advice service from 10AM–12.30PM and 1.30PM–5PM Monday to Friday on the number given above.

NAPA
5 Tavistock Place
London WC1H 9SN
Tel. 020 7383 5757
The National Association for Providers of Activities for Older People (NAPA) provides information, advice and training about activities in homes.

Pets as Therapy
Rocky Bank
6 New Road
Ditton
Kent ME20 6AD
Tel. 01732 87222
PAT has over 8500 registered PAT dogs and owners who visit hospitals, hospices and nursing and residential homes. (Enclose a 9 in × 6 in stamped self-addressed envelope.)

The Cinnamon Trust
Foundry House
Foundry Square
Hayle
Cornwall TR27 4HH
Tel. 01736 757900
The Cinnamon Trust aims to enable owners to continue to care for their pets. It provides a national fostering service so that pets can be cared for when their owners are in hospital or are unwell. If

a person is unable to care for a pet because of infirmity or acute illness, the trust volunteers can help with all aspects of pet care including walking the dog. The trust provides sanctuary to pets while their owner is in long or short-term care. The owner receives visits and regular photos and letters informing them how their pet is. There are no charges for services though donations are welcome. Send a large stamped, self-addressed envelope.

Age Exchange Reminiscence Centre
11 Blackheath Village
London SE3 9LA
Tel. 020 8318 3504
The Age Exchange Reminiscence Centre has a museum and shop and offers training in reminiscence therapy.

Winslow Press
Telford Road
Bicester
Oxford OX6 0TS
Tel. 0800 243 755
E-mail: info@winslow-press.co.uk
website: www.winslow-press.co.uk
Winslow Press has a free catalogue full of books, puzzles, games and music.

Further reading

Briscoe, T. (1991) *Developing an Activities Programme*. Winslow Press, Bicester (see Further information above). It is full of practical suggestions and imaginative ideas for activities.

The Relatives and Residents Association (1997) *As others See Us*. You may find this in your college or local library. It explores how residents, family, friends and staff see each other. The Relatives and Residents Association, London (see Further information above).

Ruddlesden, M. (1997) *You Can Do It*. Hawker Publications, London. Tel. 020 7720 2108. This is a guide to exercise for older people and is illustrated with lots of photographs of older people exercising. Highly recommended.

Chapter 8

Support When Moving to a New Environment

Introduction

This chapter covers the option group A units W3, W3.1 and W3.2 – 'support individuals experiencing a change in their care requirements and provision'. This unit applies to care assistants working in all care settings. It gives information to enable you to support the older person who moves into a new environment.

This chapter includes:

- Why older people need support
- Preparing for admission
- Admission to the home
- Supporting the older person on admission
- Dignity and privacy in homes
- Hospital admissions, emergency and planned
- Day surgery
- Outpatients visits
- Rehabilitation
- Respite care

Why older people need support

Few of us have any idea how distressing and worrying it is to enter a home. For us the home is our place of work and it holds no terrors for us. If we are unhappy in the home, we can always leave. Most older people are admitted to homes from hospital. In most cases, the admission to hospital was because of a sudden illness or accident. In other cases, the older person may have been admitted to hospital because an existing condition, such as arthritis or Parkinson's disease, became much worse. When people go to hospital, they expect to have an operation or treatment, get better and go home. It can be a terrible shock for the older person to be told that she must leave hospital but cannot go home.

Most older people given a choice would avoid homes and would prefer to return to their own homes. People entering homes may have moved from their own home to hospital, had treatment and may have been moved to another ward before entering the home. The individual may dread the thought of another move and may worry about the staff. Will they be friendly and kind? Will I get the help I need? What is it going to be like?

You need to be aware of the fears and anxieties that people will experience when entering a home. A little time and trouble taken in getting to know the individual and offering support will help allay the person's fears.

Preparing for admission

Many homes encourage residents to bring items from home to make their room seem like home. Many older people have framed photographs of their families that they treasure. The individual's family can bring in framed photographs and pictures from home and these can be hung on hooks on walls. Ornaments brought from home can be placed around the room. The individual may have a favourite chair, cushions and footstool. These could be placed in the room. Some individuals may wish to bring in other items of furniture such as small tables, a bed, wardrobe, china cabinet or bureau. If the individual can bring treasured items to the home, it becomes more like moving home than being 'put in a home'. Some individuals may wish to bring bedspreads or bed-covers from home.

Most homes have fully furnished rooms but there is no reason why this furniture cannot be stored so that the individual can bring in her own belongings. Older people who become involved in planning the move to a home, and who can decide which items to bring with them, normally feel more positive about entering the home. Some homes do not allow people to bring in furniture and bedding because they fear that the fire officer will not allow this. In homes mattresses and all soft furnishings have to meet specific fire retardancy standards. These regulations and guidelines were introduced to make homes as safe as possible. They were not, however, introduced to prevent elderly people from bringing treasured items from home. Most fire officers, if asked about this, state that the home must *purchase* items that meet fire retardancy standards and that individuals may bring items from home that do not meet these standards.

It is important to prepare the room for the person's arrival. Make sure fresh water and a glass are supplied. Check that the bed is made neatly and there are towels available. If the room appears stuffy air it, remembering to close the window a few hours before the person is expected if it is cold outside. If it is cold check that the heating is on. Make sure that the lights and the call bell work; if not, arrange repairs quickly. Check that the wardrobe has hangers in it and that the drawers and locker are clean. If possible, place a flowering plant or some flowers in the room. The person will find that the room is warm, comfortable and welcoming when she arrives. This makes a real difference; first impressions count. The impression you want to give is that the person is welcome and that you have taken the trouble to prepare for her arrival.

Admission to the home

Most older people are admitted to homes from hospitals and are transferred to the home by ambulance. The individual may have waited either on the ward or in the hospital transport department for many hours before commencing the journey to the home. In some ambulances a number of people are transported at once so the journey may take some time. By the time the older person arrives at the home her bladder may be full to bursting and she may be tired, hungry, thirsty or in pain. You should be sensitive to these possibilities; now is not the time to introduce her to all the other residents or launch into lengthy admission procedures. Introducing yourself and helping the person to her room is best. When the person's immediate needs have been met, the admission procedures can begin. If the person is very tired, she may wish to rest for a few hours first.

On first name terms?

These days people often use first names even when addressing people they do not know well. The people admitted to homes come from a different generation. They were, in their youth, addressed by their title and surname in many situations and first names were used only by close friends and family. Some older people view the way we use first names now as refreshing and friendly; others may think it over-familiar or patronising. We address children by their first names but use titles and surnames as a mark of respect. It is important to ask the individual how he or she wishes to be addressed and to use that form of address. The person who wishes to be addressed as Mrs Harley-Smith may in time ask staff to call her Ellen. Some older people, like younger people, dislike their names and use a nickname or a completely different first name. Mrs Dorothy Mason for example may be called Anne by her friends. You should make a note in the care plan or inform senior staff of how the person prefers to be addressed.

Supporting the individual after admission

People entering the home normally require a lot of help and support in the first month of admission. It takes time for the person to settle in and discover how the home is run. Care should revolve around the individual. The individual, though, will need a little time and some guidance to develop a routine that suits his or her needs. Most people develop routines in their lives and people living in homes are no different. A routine offers structure to the day but should be flexible enough to enable the individual to enjoy life.

The person entering the home has to learn a great deal: the names of the staff, mealtimes, arrangements for laundry, when activities take place. If the individual is given too much information at once, it can be difficult to remember it all. It is also difficult to decide which information is the most important. To the keen reader the location of the library books is very important, whilst to another individual that is of minor interest. Make sure that new residents and their families are aware that they can ask for information about the home.

Many homes now produce information books that provide a great deal of information about the home. These are usually made up of loose-leaf sheets held in plastic sleeves in a ring binder. Information can be updated quickly and easily. Such information books are a proposed requirement under the new national required standards. The new resident can read through the information book and find the information that is important to him or her. Some homes have produced a tape cassette giving information about the home for residents who are no longer able to read.

Dignity and privacy

One of the things many older people fear most on entering a home is the loss of dignity and privacy. At home the older person's privacy was protected by her front door; before anyone could enter, she had to open it. In homes, some rooms do not have locks. Disabilities may prevent the older person from locking her room door in other homes. Imagine what it must be like to have people barging into your room without knocking. In some homes room doors are not even closed and the older person can be seen by anyone walking along the corridor. You should always knock and ask permission before entering a person's room.

Some residents, especially those living in nursing homes, are more disabled than others. Some disabled people depend on staff to get clothing from wardrobes and chests of drawers. You should always ask the person's permission before getting clothing and items out. Some residents do not always close bedroom doors before undressing. Others forget to close the toilet door before using the toilet. It is important to be alert to such problems and to protect the person's dignity at all times.

Sharing rooms

Fifteen years ago, most people living in homes shared a room with one or two others. This was considered a great advance on geriatric hospitals where people were cared for in wards with an average of 21 beds. Now three quarters of all people living in nursing and residential homes have their own room. In some homes, patients do not have their own room but share the room with one or more people. The individual may have been living alone for many years and may be very embarrassed about sharing a room with others. The individual may have developed a close friendship with her roommate. Whatever the circumstance you should be very careful to safeguard the person's privacy and dignity in such situations. In sharing rooms, each bed has bed curtains. These should be used to protect the person's privacy when she is washing, dressing, using a commode or bedpan, or wishes to have them drawn. If the room has a washbasin, this will also have curtains. These should be used to maintain the person's privacy when washing.

Hospital admission

People living in homes are more acutely ill than before and the number of people being re-admitted to hospital from homes has risen rapidly. Older people living in residential homes are more likely to be re-admitted to hospitals than those living in nursing homes. There are three different types of admission: emergency admission, planned admission, and day surgery.

Emergency admissions

Emergency admissions are, of course, unplanned. The older person may have fallen and a fracture is suspected, or she may have become acutely ill and require hospital treatment. There is no time to prepare for the admission and the person who has settled into the home suddenly has to cope with the stress of returning to hospital. The individual is often worried about her health and the prospect of leaving the home and returning to hospital. If the person is very ill there is little time to prepare and often there is only time to prepare a toilet bag.

In emergencies, patients are taken to the accident and emergency department (A&E) where they are assessed and investigated and the doctors decide if the person requires hospital treatment. If the person's GP has arranged the emergency admission, the GP will write a letter to the medical staff in A&E. Sometimes the staff at the home have called for an ambulance and the patient has not been seen by a GP. In these circumstances, the person in charge of the home will write a letter giving details of the person's medical history, the current problem and details of any medicines that the individual is taking.

It is good practice for staff from the home to escort to hospital any patient requiring emergency treatment. In nursing homes, if the person is seriously ill a registered nurse will accompany the patient, if staffing levels allow. In smaller homes and in residential homes, care assistants may accompany an acutely ill person to hospital. Each emergency ambulance is fully equipped and has two trained paramedical staff. Both are specially trained in caring for acutely ill people. Your role is to reassure and support the individual and to communicate with hospital staff on arrival at the hospital.

Hospital accident and emergency departments can be very busy. You should stay with the older person, accompany her to X-ray if required, explain procedures, and provide practical help and moral support. Sometimes people remain in accident and emergency for twelve or more hours while hospital staff try to find a vacant bed. Waits of 24 hours or more are not uncommon especially in the winter months. You may have to telephone the home for advice if there are delays in admission. When the individual is admitted to the ward, you should remain until the person is settled in if possible. Find out as much as possible about the plan of treatment before leaving. If possible, try to get some indication of how long the person is expected to remain in hospital.

Keeping in touch
Approximately 10% of people living in homes have no close relatives or friends. Although it is important to keep in touch with all patients who are in hospital, those without family or friends may feel particularly alone and lost and require special support. A daily telephone call to check how the individual is progressing, and to leave a message for them, will help the person feel she is not forgotten. If possible visit the person in hospital, telephoning first to check if she requires anything from home.

Many older people worry that if they become ill or require greater levels of care than before, the home will refuse to have them back.

Residential homes do not normally employ registered nurses and employ fewer staff than nursing homes. In some cases if the older person becomes more disabled she may be unable to return to the residential home. Most nursing homes care for older people who require high levels of skilled care, but some are unable to care for people with very high dependency needs. It is important to find out what level of care is provided within the home. If an individual is worried that she will be unable to return to the home, inform your manager. The manager can visit, discuss this with the person, and in the vast majority of cases set the person's mind at rest.

People returning to the home after a hospital stay may be weaker and less able to care for themselves than previously. It may take time for the individual to regain strength and ability after an illness. The person's room should be prepared ready for re-admission and any get well cards from friends, relatives, residents and staff put in the room.

Planned admissions

In the past older people in homes were seldom re-admitted to hospital for non-emergency treatment. Now, though, attitudes are more positive and medical staff are more aware that in some cases hospital treatment may improve an older person's quality of life. Planned hospital treatment is becoming more common.

When non-emergency treatment is required, there is time to prepare and support the person. You should find out as much as possible about treatment planned. Normally hospital and professional staff working in homes explain the treatment in detail; however, residents may wish to discuss treatment with you. You may need professional advice about planned treatment.

Day surgery

Day surgery is becoming very common. Now people who a few years ago would have remained in hospital for a few days after surgery are admitted in the morning and discharged home in the evening. It is possible to treat greater numbers of people on a day surgery basis. Many older people who develop cataracts find that instead of joining long waiting lists they can be treated quickly as day cases.

People requiring day surgery are normally sent by their GP to see a specialist at the local hospital. If the specialist feels that the case is suitable, the person is placed on a day surgery waiting list. A short time before planned admission (usually a week) the person visits the day surgery unit for assessment and investigation, and professional staff give full details of the planned surgery and the care required afterwards. Most surgery units supply written patient information booklets.

On the day of the operation, if a general anaesthetic is required the person does not eat or drink. (The day surgery unit will supply instructions about eating and drinking.) Many cases of day surgery are carried out under local anaesthetic. The person is normally admitted to the ward in the morning, prepared for surgery, and taken to theatre. After the operation the patient usually rests for some time, nursing staff carry out routine post-operative checks and the doctor examines the patient before agreeing discharge if all is well.

It is policy in most homes that a member of staff accompanies the individual to hospital and remains at the hospital providing support and practical help during the person's stay. If you are to escort a patient to day surgery and wish to watch the operation discuss this with your manager. The nurse in charge of the day surgery unit can ask the surgeon if you can enter the theatre and observe the operation. Many surgeons explain the operation as they carry it out. Many older people become increasingly worried about day surgery as the day of the operation approaches. Knowing that a member of staff will be with them makes many people less anxious.

Outpatient visits

Visits to the hospital outpatient department may be required for a number of reasons:

- Following surgery at the hospital
- To check on an existing medical condition
- To consider if further treatment is required for a specific problem

In some homes, all older people are escorted to outpatient's appointments by a member of staff. In other homes, transport is arranged to hospital but the home does not provide an escort. In some cases, a member of the resident's family arranges to meet her at the hospital. Almost all nursing homes provide escorts, while the policy in residential homes varies.

If you are asked to escort an older person to an outpatient's appointment, make sure that you know the reason for the visit. Is it a routine check-up? Is it to discuss possible further treatment? The individual or your manager will have an appointment card giving details of which clinic to attend, the doctor to be seen and the time of the appointment. Senior staff may also send a letter giving details of current medication and treatment.

If ambulance transport has been arranged it is important to bear in mind that ambulances can arrive very much earlier or later than ordered. Help the person get ready in plenty of time. An early breakfast or lunch may be required. When transport arrives, it may be picking up a number of other people before going to the hospital. Ask the individual if she wishes to use the toilet before leaving. If it is cold outside make sure the individual's coat is at hand and help her to put it on before leaving.

You may find that you have to wait a few hours in outpatients before the patient is seen, so be prepared. Take some 20p pieces so that you can both have a cup of tea while waiting; most outpatients departments have vending machines. Take extra change so that you can telephone the home if there is a problem getting transport back. Take something to pass the time; perhaps magazines, the person's knitting or some playing cards. When the doctor sees the patient check that you both understand the outcome of the visit. On returning to the home the individual may be feeling tired after the journey. Be sensitive to her needs and offer the opportunity to rest if she wishes. Inform the person in charge of the outcome of the visit.

Rehabilitation

Greater numbers of old people are now admitted to homes so that they can fully recover from operation or illness and return home. If the individual is admitted to the home for a short stay, you will normally work with a range of other staff to help prepare the person for discharge home. Many staff, such as the physiotherapist and occupational therapist, and the GP will be working with the person to help her to regain the ability to care for herself at home. Your role is an important one. It is to work with the team. Recovering after a major illness is hard work, and there will be times when the older person feels low. You can offer encouragement and support at such times.

Respite care

There are seven million people caring for older people in their own homes in the UK. They care for relatives or friends who would otherwise require long-term care. For many years, carers have not received the help required to enable them to continue to care. Now respite care is becoming more available and homes will be caring for more people on a respite basis in the next few years.

Respite care is a planned period of care. The older person is admitted to the home for a short period, normally two weeks on a regular basis, so that the carer can have a break. Caring for an older person at home without assistance is very hard work. Many carers find it difficult to do the things that we take for granted, such as go to the shops or visit friends. The aim of respite care is to enable carers to continue caring for longer periods by offering planned breaks.

In homes a number of beds are booked as respite beds. The individual is booked in for certain weeks throughout the year. Many older people who are admitted for respite care for the first time worry that they will never return home. You should be sensitive to such fears and reassure individuals that this is a temporary admission. Many carers have developed ways of meeting the older person's needs at home and have developed a routine. It is important that staff obtain as much information as possible about the older person's normal care and routine and do not disrupt this. It may be easier for two members of staff to help the person onto the toilet, but if the carer and the older person live alone and have been managing, you will only make life more difficult when the older person returns home. If the person's bedroom at home is upstairs, staff should be careful to continue walking upstairs with the older person and not use the lift. If the older person loses the ability to walk upstairs, how will she cope at home?

During the period of respite, care staff may be able to help organise services such as chiropody or suggest that aids such as grab rails may help the older person manage at home. Such suggestions and offers of help should be made sensitively as carers may feel that staff are critical of their ability to cope. Many older people and their carers benefit from regular respite care and find that the support of staff in the early days is vitally important.

Summary

The role of homes is changing rapidly. Now older people move from hospital to home and home to hospital more than ever before. Change is difficult to cope with at the best of times. Older people who have been ill or who have undergone recent surgery can feel very vulnerable and worried as they move between care environments. Care assistants who are aware of older people's worries can respond sensitively and help individuals adjust to changing circumstances.

Portfolio preparation

 Your assessor must have evidence that you can meet the performance criteria for this unit. Before beginning the units discuss assessment strategies with your assessor. Most of the evidence for this unit can be gained by direct observation of your work. However often residents hesitate to ask questions when someone else (your assessor) is present. You may be asked to provide the following types of evidence.

- Products. This might include details of an information leaflet you have produced. One NVQ student prepared an information package about cataract surgery for a resident.
- Witness testimony. This is a statement from a senior member of staff, a relative or a resident. This might be a statement detailing how you have helped support a resident moving to the home or a resident admitted for respite care. Remember to ask a senior member of staff before asking a relative or resident for a witness testimony. This will seldom be a problem but it is a matter of courtesy. The statement could be recorded on a tape if the person is unable to write. It could be dictated, written down, and witnessed by a senior member of staff.
- Written work. You might be asked to prepare a piece of work about how you help residents to feel that the home is their home. You might be asked to write a case history on how you helped a resident settle in. You might be asked to outline how you use the home's policy on admission, any difficulties you have faced and how you have dealt with them.

Your assessor will also use other methods to help you gain evidence for this unit. These may include:

- Verbal questioning
- Written questions

Role-play may be used. Your assessor may use role-play and simulations to check that you have the ability to put theory into practice.

Further reading

Alzheimer's Disease Society (1993) *Deprivation & Dementia*. A report by the Alzheimer's Disease Society, London. This report discusses the resources needed to help carers continue to provide care. It gives a series of case studies that illustrate the difficulties that carers face when caring for a relative at home.

Carers National Association (1993) *Listening to Carers*. Carers National Association, London. This book discusses the services that carers need to help them continue to care for relatives at home.

Chapter 9

Mobility

Introduction

This chapter covers the option group A units Z6, Z6.1, Z6.2 – 'enable clients to maintain and improve their mobility'. The option group B units Z5, Z5.1, Z5.2 Z5.3 – 'enable clients to maintain their mobility and make journeys and visits' – are also covered.

This chapter provides information on:

- The benefits of remaining mobile
- How illness affects mobility
- The dangers of immobility
- Helping older people to remain mobile
- Walking aids
- Helping and encouraging older people to use aids
- Obtaining aids
- Helping people to maintain independence in wheelchairs
- Transferring from a wheelchair
- Exercise and passive movement
- Assisting people to prepare for journeys and visits
- Accompanying people on journeys and visits

Benefits of remaining mobile

The ability to move around freely is one of the most basic of human rights. It is an ability that we often take for granted. Many older people who enter homes have problems moving around. Some are unable to move unaided from bed to chair and some are bedbound. Some develop deformities that mean that they can no longer straighten arms or legs, and hands may become permanently closed in fists.

Some professional staff in some homes may tell you that such changes are the inevitable effects of ageing and that older people become immobile because of ageing. Whilst older people may become immobile in the last few months or weeks of life, many older people living in nursing and residential homes become immobile because of poorly managed care. *It does not have to be this way.*

The way staff work within homes may not only prevent some older people from regaining mobility after illness, it can also cause older people to become less mobile and more dependent. The goal of care in nursing and residential homes should be to enable older people to retain and regain mobility. This in turn enables them to retain the ability to care for themselves and enjoy a superior quality of life within the home. It also reduces staff workload.

This chapter will outline how illness affects the older person's ability to move around, the dangers of immobility, and how carers can help older people to retain independence after illness. Some older people, normally those who are extremely ill or disabled, will require greater levels of assistance and may need to be moved. This is dealt with in Chapter 10.

How illness affects an older person's ability to move around

Many older people are admitted to nursing and residential homes from hospital, although some are admitted from home. Most are admitted because the effects of an accident or illness mean that the individual can no longer manage to care for him or herself at home. Some older people are admitted because a long-standing illness has worsened and it is impossible to provide the levels of support and care required at home. Others are admitted because of a sudden illness or an accident.

It is possible for many older people who are unable to care for themselves at home to enjoy life in a home where the support they require is given. There is a danger that staff who are not aware of the older person's abilities may discourage the older person from moving around the home. In other cases, older people may require encouragement, help, support and aids to help them walk. It is important that you understand how illness affects an individual's ability to walk, so that you can offer appropriate support and help.

Arthritis

Arthritis is a disease that affects all people as they age. Adults start to develop arthritic changes from the age of 40 onwards. Although all older people have arthritis, not all suffer the symptoms. Approximately 12% of men and 25% of women over the age of 70 suffer pain, stiffness and difficulties in moving because of arthritis. There are two types of arthritis: osteo-arthritis and rheumatoid arthritis.

Osteo-arthritis

Osteo means bone, and arthritis means damage or inflammation. Osteo-arthritis is damage and inflammation to the bone. The ends of bone at joints are covered with a thin layer of smooth material called cartilage. The end of the bone and the cartilage are surrounded by a thick fluid that is called synovial fluid. This is contained in a thin membrane that is known as the synovial membrane. Cartilage and synovial fluid cushion the end of the bone from the effects of movement and act as shock absorbers. The cartilage becomes thinned and roughened when osteo-arthritis is present. The bone is not so well protected from the shock of movement and thickens, the amount of fluid increases and the joint appears swollen. In severe osteo-arthritis, the cartilage can wear away completely and bone can rub on bone. The joints affected usually become visibly deformed. Figure 9.1 shows a healthy knee joint and Figure 9.2 shows a knee joint affected by osteo-arthritis.

The causes of osteo-arthritis are not yet known. People are more likely to develop osteo-arthritis as they become older and people who have injured a joint or had an operation on a joint are

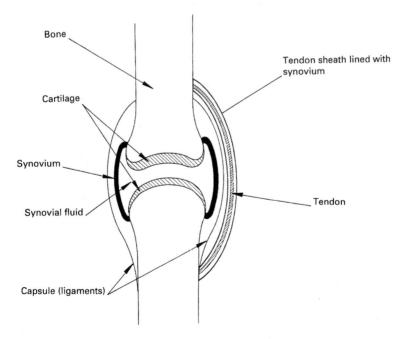

Bone

Tendon sheath lined with synovium

Cartilage

Synovium

Tendon

Synovial fluid

Capsule (ligaments)

Fig. 9.1 A healthy knee joint.

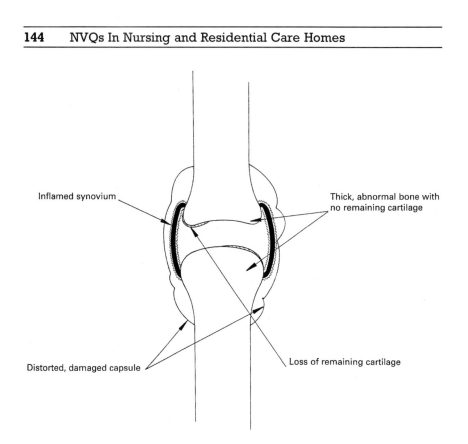

Inflamed synovium

Thick, abnormal bone with
no remaining cartilage

Distorted, damaged capsule

Loss of remaining cartilage

Fig. 9.2 An arthritic knee joint.

more likely to develop osteo-arthritis. It often develops in people
who have taken part in active sports.

The joints affected are usually the hand, hips, knees and big
toes. Osteo-arthritis of the hip usually affects one hip more
severely than the other. It can lead to one leg becoming slightly
shorter. This can cause walking difficulties and back pain. Osteo-
arthritis of the hip is more common in men than in women. Osteo-
arthritis of the knee is more common in women.

Osteo-arthritis normally affects only one or two joints. Although
many people who suffer from osteo-arthritis find that pain and
stiffness is worse in damp weather, dampness does not cause the
problem. People all over the world suffer from this condition.

Osteo-arthritis causes pain, stiffness and swelling. The stiffness
is made worse by remaining in one position for a long time, and
will improve after a few minutes exercise. Pain is normally treated
by pain killing tablets, known as analgesics. Aspirin and paracetamol are commonly prescribed by doctors. If these are not
effective, anti-inflammatory drugs are often prescribed. These
drugs act not only by treating pain but also by reducing the
inflammation in the joint. Such drugs are known as non-steroidal

anti-inflammatory drugs. Neurofen, a popular painkiller that can be bought over the counter, is a non-steroidal anti-inflammatory drug.

Overweight people who suffer from osteo-arthritis will feel much better if they lose weight, because extra weight increases the strain on joints.

Rheumatoid arthritis

Rheumatoid arthritis is an inflammatory disease of the joints. The synovial tissue that covers the joints becomes inflamed. This causes the affected joints to become hot, swollen and painful. Figure 9.3 shows how rheumatoid arthritis affects a joint.

Rheumatoid arthritis normally affects many joints. A person with rheumatoid arthritis may suffer from pain and inflammation in the shoulders, arms, wrists, fingers and toes. Although this is a chronic disease, there are often periods when it settles down and causes few problems. At other times the individual suffers an acute attack and joints become very painful. During an acute attack, people are advised to rest the joints as much as possible.

In mild cases, paracetamol or aspirin are prescribed. In more severe cases, non-steroidal anti-inflammatory drugs are

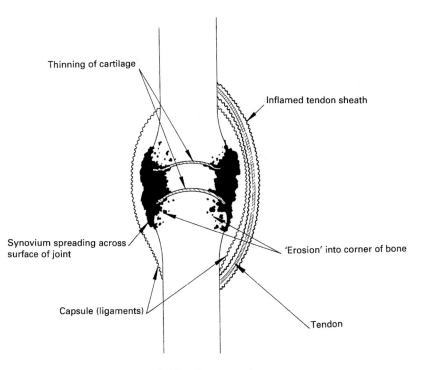

Fig. 9.3   How rheumatoid arthritis affects a joint.

prescribed. Doctors may prescribe steroids in severe cases. The cause of rheumatoid arthritis is not yet known.

Benefits of exercise

It is important that people suffering from all types of arthritis keep as active as possible. Many years ago it was thought that the best treatment for all types was rest. Many people with arthritis of all types were admitted to hospital and kept on strict bedrest. Arthritic joints were often put in plaster of Paris casts to prevent any movement. It was thought then that joints became worn out by too much movement. Now people who are suffering from acute rheumatoid arthritis are advised to rest their swollen joints but to take gentle exercise. People suffering from chronic rheumatoid arthritis and osteo-arthritis are advised to carry on with gentle exercise and remain as mobile as possible.

Some older people worry that exercise will cause further damage to joints and need reassurance that this will not happen. Gentle exercise will reduce stiffness and help them to remain as fit as possible.

Further information

The Arthritis and Rheumatism Council for Research (ARC)
Copeman House
St Mary's Court
Chesterfield
Derbyshire S41 7TD
Tel. 01246 558033
ARC is a charity that provides information for patients, carers, doctors and nurses. It produces a wide range of leaflets and booklets, including *Rheumatoid Arthritis* – a handbook for patients, and *Osteo-Arthritis* – a booklet for patients. Single copies are available free of charge. ARC will provide full details of their publications on request.

Strokes

Many older people are admitted to homes after suffering from strokes. The medical term for a stroke is a cerebro-vascular accident. Nursing and medical staff often refer to this as a CVA. Normally blood flows around the brain, feeding it with oxygen and sugar (Fig. 9.4). A stroke causes the blood supply to the brain to be interrupted and part of the brain is starved of oxygen.

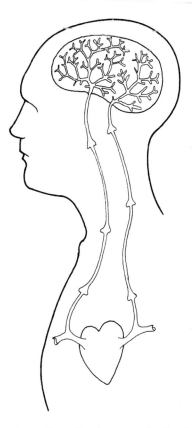

Fig. 9.4 Blood flows from the heart to the brain via the arterial circulation.

There are two main causes of strokes. Some occur because the blood becomes too thick; blood cells stick together and form a clot, which prevents blood reaching an area of the brain (Fig. 9.5a). In other cases the blood vessels supplying the brain leak and bleed into the brain (Fig. 9.5b). In both cases, the blood supply to the brain is interrupted and the brain becomes damaged. The amount of damage a stroke causes varies enormously. The longer the person is unconscious after a stroke, the greater the damage. Once an area of the brain has been damaged, it cannot recover (Fig. 9.6). It is estimated that we use only about a tenth of our brain and often other parts of the brain learn to do the job of the damaged area.

People who have suffered from strokes often develop weakness or paralysis down one side of their body. A weakness is known as hemi-pareisis and paralysis as hemiplegia. Many older people who suffer from strokes can regain movement and continue to recover for up to two years after a stroke. Some older people remain

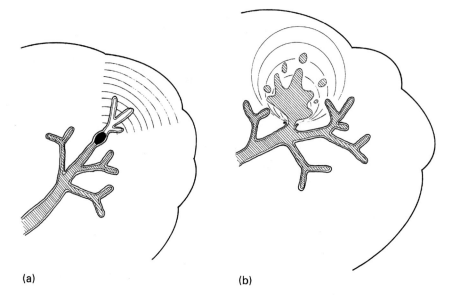

(a)   (b)

Fig. 9.5 (a) A clot lodged in one of the articles in the brain; (b) a ruptured blood vessel.

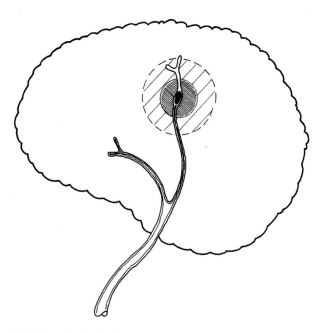

Fig. 9.6 The dark shading shows the area of brain tissue which no longer functions because of the stroke. The circled area with diagonal line shading is the brain tissue affected by bruising and swelling. This part of the brain will recover.

paralysed down one side but can learn to walk with special aids. Others can learn to move around freely in wheelchairs and transfer from wheelchair to chair, bed or toilet. You can help people to regain as much independence as possible following a stroke by encouraging them to exercise and to learn how to cope with disability and remain as independent as possible.

Further information

The Stroke Association
CHSA House
Whitecross Street
London EC1 8JJ
Tel. 020 7490 2686
The Stroke Association is the only national charity concerned solely with stroke. The Association provides telephone help-lines and offers support to over 400 stroke clubs. It funds research into the causes of stroke and aims to educate the public in how to remain healthy and reduce the risk of stroke. A number of leaflets are available free, including information on transient ischaemic attacks, physiotherapy and occupational therapy. A number of booklets, books and videos are also available.

Fractures

Older people are more at risk of falling than younger people. As people age the bones become thinner and weaker and more likely to break or fracture. This is because of a disease called osteoporosis that is especially common in women.

When older people fall, they often break wrists, thigh bones (femurs) or hips. Nowadays most people who suffer from fractured femurs have surgical treatment. The bone is pulled together and held in place with a metal plate and screws. If the neck of the femur is fractured a screw may be inserted to hold the bone together, or the surgeon may replace the neck of the femur with metal. If the hip is fractured, the surgeon may carry out a hip replacement.

Many older people who have fallen over, broken a bone and undergone major surgery are discharged to homes unable to walk. This may be because the individual is in a lot of pain following treatment. Carers should ask such individuals if they are in pain and inform professional staff so that painkillers may be given. Some older people who are in pain do not tell staff. One survey carried out in hospital found that patients who were in pain waited for nursing staff to ask about pain because they did not want to appear to be complaining. The same survey found that nursing staff waited for patients to tell them that they were in pain. You should learn to observe individuals, as often our behaviour shows whether we are in pain. If you think the person is in pain, ask.

Many older people who have had a severe fall have lost all confidence in walking. They may require encouragement and help in beginning to walk again. Some older people who have had surgery to repair a fractured femur or hip may now have one leg shorter than the other. This can make walking difficult and dangerous. Fortunately, it can easily be corrected by ordering and providing special shoes. One shoe has a slightly higher, built-up heel and this corrects any differences in leg length. Further details are given later in the chapter.

Vision

Poor vision can make it difficult for older people to move around freely. Research from the Royal College of Opticians shows that 96% of people over the age of 80 require spectacles. Many older people admitted to nursing and residential homes wear spectacles but may not have had their eyes tested for many years. New spectacles and an up to date prescription for lenses may help them to move around with newfound confidence.

Some older people suffer from cataracts. These affect vision long before they are visible to carers. Now many older people can benefit from cataract surgery. An eye test will detect the presence of cataracts.

Some older people suffer from eye diseases such as glaucoma. Untreated glaucoma can cause blindness. An eye test will detect the presence of glaucoma and the person's doctor can prescribe eye drops which will prevent vision deteriorating.

Recently doctors carried out research to find out why people admitted to hospital with falls had fallen. They found that most of the people who had fallen had very poor vision. Almost all visual problems could be treated.

Some older people suffer from extremely poor vision and little can be done to improve it. If staff are aware that the individual's vision is poor, they can ensure that the environment is as safe as possible. Details of maintaining a safe environment are given in Chapter 3.

The dangers of immobility

When older people lose the ability to move around freely, it has a devastating effect on their physical and mental health.

Many older people fear becoming a burden and wish to carry on caring for themselves. The idea of being dependent on others can be very upsetting. Imagine what it must be like to be unable to walk to the toilet and to have to rely on others to take you. Imagine how it must feel to be unable to get up when you wish or to go to bed when you wish. Many older people become depressed, anxious and upset when they lose the ability to move around.

The physical effects of immobility are also distressing. People who sit for long periods often find that their feet and ankles become swollen. This is because they are not walking. Walking helps the veins to return blood to the heart. People who are sitting for long periods are at risk of developing blood clots in the legs. These are called deep vein thrombosis. A deep vein thrombosis can break away from the vein in the leg and enter the venous circulation. The clot then travels around the body until it becomes stuck either in a heart valve or in the vein entering the lung (pulmonary vein). This condition is known as a pulmonary embolism and can be fatal.

Moving around causes us to breathe more deeply and this deep breathing is one of the things which protects us against chest infections. People who are immobile are more at risk of developing a chest infection than those who walk around.

Movement causes the bowel to contract. People who do not move around are more at risk of becoming constipated. People who can go to the toilet without help are less likely to suffer from incontinence than those who require help. People who require help are dependent on staff to take them to the toilet. Often staff do not respond quickly enough to an individual's call for assistance (perhaps because they are doing something else) and incontinence can result. People who are not using muscles find that their muscles quickly become smaller and weaker and strength and ability is rapidly lost.

Helping older people to move around

The role of care assistants in helping individuals to retain or regain independence is important. You can help or hinder the older person who wishes to remain independent. The care assistant who 'takes over' and offers or insists on doing things for the person who can do it themselves is not helping and making things easier for the person. The care assistant is making life more difficult. Faced with such 'help' some older people can feel that there is little point in trying and that it is better to let the staff 'get on with it'.

Care assistants can unintentionally make older people feel useless. If you offer to bring a person downstairs in a wheelchair 'because it's quicker', the person may soon lose the confidence and strength to come down alone. She will also lose independence and may begin to feel that she is a nuisance and a burden to staff. The sensitive carer will provide support and help without robbing the person of her independence.

Case history

Mrs Edna Brown has lived in a nursing home for some time. At the morning report staff are informed that she fell while walking to bed the night before. The care assistant caring for her, Sarah Easton, asks Mrs Brown how she feels. Mrs Brown confesses that she feels shaken by her fall. Sarah offers to help her get her clothes ready and asks if she would like any help with washing or dressing. Mrs Brown says she can manage. Later Sarah walks with Mrs Brown to the lounge. This action gives Mrs Brown confidence; help is at hand if needed but Mrs Brown has maintained her independence.

Walking aids

Many older people rely on walking aids to help them move around. Some older people are admitted to homes with aids. Some individuals who do not have aids might be able to move around independently or with less help if they had an aid. There are several different types of walking aid. The commonest is the Zimmer or walking frame.

Zimmer frames

Zimmer frames (Fig. 9.7a) help older people who are unsteady on their feet or who lack confidence, because when they are used properly people are more stable. Zimmer frames come in a variety of heights and widths; it is possible to adjust the height on some frames. Each person is measured for his or her frame so that it is the right height. Too tall a frame encourages an individual to reach up; this unbalances the person and can cause falls. Too low a frame can lead to a person bending over the frame, which can also cause falls. When an older person has been measured for a frame, it is important to label the frame so that frames do not become mixed up. This is an important safety measure if falls are to be prevented.

Zimmer frames have small rubber ends on each of the four legs, called ferrules. Each ferrule should have a whorl-like pattern on it. These patterns of raised rubber prevent the frame from slipping. You should check every few months that the patterns have not worn off as worn ferrules can lead to the frame slipping and the individual falling. Ferrules can be replaced if this happens, new ones being obtained from the community supplies department of the local NHS community trust.

Some older people, especially those suffering from arthritis, do not have the strength to lift a frame off the ground and are unable to use Zimmer frames. They are often supplied with special Zimmer frames that have wheels at the bottom (Fig. 9.7b). The individual pushes the wheeled frame along. Wheeled frames are normally supplied after a careful assessment. An older person who tends to move quickly could easily fall or injure themselves using a wheeled frame. The wheels of these frames require oiling from time to time.

Gutter frames

Gutter frames are specialist frames. They are often supplied to individuals who have difficulty in gripping and lifting a normal frame (Fig.9.8). Such frames are often supplied to individuals who

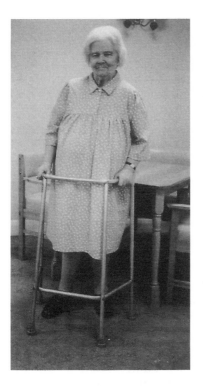

(a)   (b)

Fig. 9.7   (a) Zimmer frame; (b) wheeled Zimmer frame.

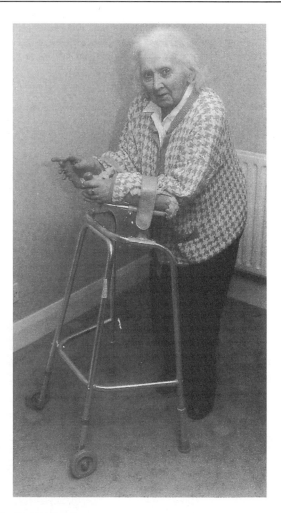

Fig. 9.8 Gutter frame.

have severe arthritis in the arms and hands. Such individuals may require help to stand up and gain their balance on the gutter frame.

Tripods

Tripods are often used as walking aids by individuals who have suffered from strokes. The stroke may have left the individual with a weakness or paralysis on one side, which means that using a Zimmer frame is not possible. Tripods should be fitted to ensure that they are the correct height. A person with a left-sided weakness will require a right handed tripod and one with a right-sided weakness a left-handed tripod. Some tripods have a handle that can be swivelled around to accommodate right and left-handed users. Using a tripod allows the individual to improve balance and regain as much independence as possible. Sometimes people are able to walk alone using a tripod after a stroke; sometimes they need someone to help (Fig. 9.9).

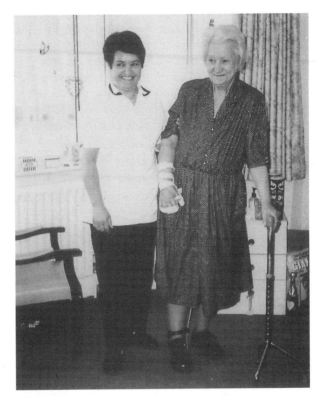

Fig. 9.9   Care assistant helping an individual to use a tripod.

Walking sticks

When older people feel unsteady, they often buy walking sticks. It is important that walking sticks are the correct height for the individual and do not encourage stretching or stooping, which can lead to falls. Unfortunately, few older people are measured for walking sticks. If an individual enters the home with walking sticks and these appear to be the wrong height, the height should be checked. Further details are given later in the chapter.

How aids are obtained

Many older people enter homes with aids. These may have been supplied in hospital or at home. You may feel that an older person might benefit from a walking aid. Sometimes an older person is no longer able to manage with a particular aid. The person who managed well with a Zimmer frame but who has suffered a stroke is no longer able to use her frame. She may benefit from a tripod.

Walking aids are normally supplied by the community physiotherapist. The procedure for obtaining aids varies from area to area. Normally the patient's doctor asks the physiotherapist to see the patient and assess for a walking aid. In some areas doctors are provided with special forms that they must complete, while in others the doctor writes a letter to the physiotherapist. The physiotherapist visits and assesses the patient, then normally completes a form and orders the walking aid.

Walking aids are usually delivered direct to the home. Staff are often asked to call the physiotherapist when the aid arrives. The physiotherapist normally visits, makes any adjustments that are required, and checks that the aid is safe and suitable.

Helping and encouraging older people to use their aids

Many people are nervous when they first receive aids. You can help individuals gain confidence by encouraging them to use the aids. Older people who are getting used to an aid should be accompanied on walks until staff are sure that they can walk safely and confidently alone. Some older people who use aids will always require someone to assist them. The use of an aid in such circumstances means that the older person can walk with an aid and one carer instead of two.

People who depend on aids should always have these placed near them. It is easy to move an aid out of the way when settling someone in bed and forget to place it back within reach of the individual before leaving the room. If someone is unable to reach their walking aid, they may try to get up and walk without it. This can lead to a fall and the older person could suffer from a serious injury.

Using aids enables many older people to become more independent than before. Older people who use aids benefit from the exercise involved in walking. They feel more in control and are less likely to feel depressed. Family and friends may feel more confident about taking the individual on short outings and the individual's quality of life improves. The exercise improves the circulation to the legs and reduces the risk of swollen ankles and legs. Movement helps the bowel to work properly and the individual is less likely to become constipated. Gentle exercise such as walking may give patients who had no interest in food an appetite. Overweight patients benefit from exercise, and the ability to move around and go on outings will help them to lose weight or to avoid gaining more. Staff within the home have more time to spend chatting or taking part in activities with the patient as they no longer have to spend so much time helping the person move around.

Wheelchairs

Helping people in wheelchairs retain and regain independence

Some people, because of disability or disease, are unable to walk even with aids and must use wheelchairs to help them move around. Patients with diseases such as multiple sclerosis or severe arthritis may need wheelchairs. People who are unable to walk can still retain independence if they are helped and encouraged to do so. Unfortunately, many people are issued with wheelchairs that they cannot use themselves and they must rely on others to push them. This is a great shame as many people are able to learn how to move around in their wheelchairs. There are two different types of (non-electric) wheelchairs.

Self-propelling wheelchairs (Fig. 9.10) have large wheels, which have circular metal handgrips around them. The person uses the handgrip to turn the wheel and push herself along. Many people are able to become independent when they get used to their wheelchairs. Some people who have suffered from strokes have only one working hand with which to push the wheelchair. Some people who have had stroke request that the footplate on the side of the body not affected by the stroke is left off. The person then uses the unaffected leg to help steer and move the wheelchair around. Other wheelchairs are designed for people who are unable to move around themselves (Fig. 9.11). These chairs have smaller wheels.

Transferring

Many older people can be encouraged and helped to move around the home in wheelchairs. Although the older person has lost the ability to walk, she has retained independence and is not forced to rely on staff to move around. Moving a wheelchair around is fairly hard work and this exercise strengthens the muscles in the arms and chest. Many people who use wheelchairs can use these strong arm and chest muscles to transfer from wheelchair to chair, wheelchair to toilet or wheelchair to bed.

When transferring, the side of the wheelchair is normally removed. In some cases the individual is able to put some weight

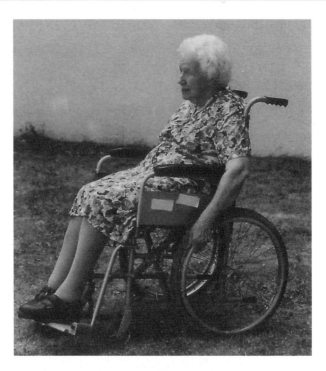

Fig. 9.10 Self-propelling wheelchair.

on their legs and slide into a chair while holding onto one side of the wheelchair and the arm of the chair. When transferring from wheelchair to toilet, grab rails can be used to pull the body up. The care assistant can, if required, pull down clothing. The person can then use the grab rails to pull themselves over and onto the toilet seat.

When transferring from bed to chair some patients use a special pole known as a 'monkey pole', which has a grip suspended from a chain. This grip helps the person to lift up and swing over into the chair. Using a monkey pole requires strong muscles and the ability to lift the arms above the head. Some people, especially those suffering from arthritis, are unable to use monkey poles. They may find using a special board (known as a transfer board) easier. One end of the board is placed on the wheelchair and the other on the bed (usually this end is placed under the mattress). The care assistant remains with the person who uses the arms and, if possible, muscles in the lower body to wiggle along the board and into the bed or chair. The board is then removed. Some people are able to transfer independently without assistance or supervision.

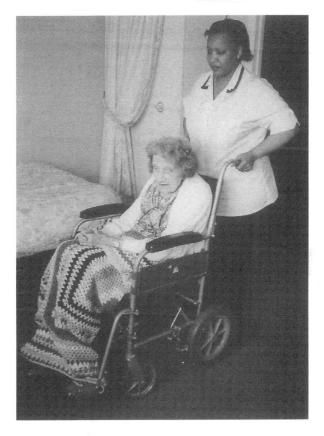

Fig. 9.11 Transit chair, non-self-propelling.

Keeping wheelchairs in good repair

Older people who rely on wheelchairs to move around need chairs that are kept in good repair. Poorly maintained wheelchairs are at best difficult to use and at worst dangerous. Tyres should be kept firm. It is very difficult to push a wheelchair with flat tyres, and flat tyres can prevent wheelchair brakes from working properly. Wheelchairs that move when someone is transferring can cause falls. All wheelchairs are supplied with a pump and tyres that are becoming soft should be pumped up. You should find out who is responsible for this in your home. Tyres that become soft again shortly after being pumped up may have a puncture. Wheelchair tyres should have a clearly visible tread on them. If the tread has worn away, the tyres need replacing.

Wheelchair brakes can easily become damaged; if the brakes are not working, urgent repairs should be organised.

Organising repairs

Wheelchairs are supplied to individuals. Each wheelchair should have the individual's name on it. When wheelchairs are supplied to individuals in homes, the manager is supplied with a reference number for each chair.

Arrangements for repair of wheelchairs vary from area to area. In some areas, the community health trust (which is responsible for supplying and maintaining the wheelchairs of people living in homes) employs its own staff to repair wheelchairs. In other areas, the community health trust employs a contractor to carry out repairs. The manager of your home will be able to tell you what the local arrangements are.

In all cases the staff responsible for carrying out repairs are telephoned. Often a message has to be left on an answerphone as staff are out repairing, collecting or delivering wheelchairs. The name of the patient, type of wheelchair and reference number, and if possible details of the fault, are required. The repairer requires these details so that spare parts, which may be required, can be brought along. If possible the chair will be repaired or parts such as tyres replaced at the home. If this is not possible the chair is taken away for repairs and a replacement chair is loaned to the person until the wheelchair can be returned.

Exercise and passive movement

You should encourage patients to exercise and to move their limbs. Sometimes, though, people are unable to do so. A person who has lost all movement and feeling in the legs because of a disease such as multiple sclerosis may not be able to move her legs. An individual who has suffered from a severe stroke may be unable to understand or remember your advice on moving his paralysed hand.

Joints that are not moved quickly stiffen up. The tendons, which connect joints, contract and shorten. Muscles become smaller and waste away. If the legs of an older person who is unable to move them are not moved, they can become fixed. A person who sits for most of the day in a wheelchair can develop legs that are fixed in a permanent sitting position. If the legs are not gently moved and exercised, it will become impossible to straighten them within a few months. These changes are known as flexion contractures. You can prevent such deformities by gently moving limbs that the person is unable to move for himself or herself. If there is any existing deformity or limbs do not move normally do not attempt to move the limbs. Seek professional advice.

Splints

Sometimes patients who have suffered from strokes are supplied with special aids, known as splints, to prevent deformities and contractures to the hand on the affected side. Splints and exercise or passive movement are used together. The splint prevents the hand from remaining in a closed position when it is not being exercised. If a patient has a splint, it is important to help put it on and encourage its use. There are several different types of hand splint. Each splint is made especially for the individual patient. A registered nurse or physiotherapist can provide advice and information.

Assisting people to prepare for journeys and visits

For most of us home is a cradle from which we spring, not a prison that encloses us. Many older people enjoy going out. Others need support and help to prepare for journeys and visits. Some people have been housebound for years before coming into the home. The outside world can seem a very hostile and threatening place to some older people. You can help the person prepare for journeys and visits by:

- Organising local trips. A visit to the nearby shops to choose toiletries or buy items is less threatening than a visit to hospital or a long trip.
- Helping the person to plan the trip
- Making sure that the person is able to manage the trip. A person who is able to walk within the home may not be able to manage a long walk. Check what the person is capable of before the trip.
- Help the person to choose suitable clothing. This not only helps ensure that the person is comfortable; it also makes the individual feel in control.

Accompanying residents on visits and journeys

There are many reasons why you might be asked to accompany a resident on a journey. Sometimes you will be escorting the person to a hospital for treatment, or you may be asked to escort the person on an outing or a family celebration.

Case history

Sidney Bashford's youngest grandchild Helen was getting married. Sidney, as head of the family, had attended all the family celebrations for over half a century but he was becoming increasingly frail. His family desperately wanted him to attend but were anxious about their ability to look after him during the wedding. They asked if Adam Odigie could accompany Sidney to the wedding. Adam encouraged Sidney to talk about any fears he had about his granddaughter's big day and did his best to plan for every eventuality.

Adam arrived early, helped Sidney to dress and prepare for the journey. Adam and Sidney travelled to the wedding by car. Adam was on hand to help meet Sidney's care needs.

Summary

Many older people admitted to homes have difficulty in moving around. Your approach and attitude are important in helping older people remain as independent as possible.

Your role is to support older people and help them to retain independence. Many older people rely on aids to move around. Some people use wheelchairs but wheelchair users can still retain independence and freedom. Some people require assistance to move paralysed limbs to prevent deformity developing. Older people living within the home have an enormous range of abilities and care assistants who understand individual needs can work as part of the team to meet those needs.

Portfolio preparation

Your assessor must have evidence that you can meet the performance criteria for these units. Before beginning these units discuss assessment strategies with your assessor. Most of the evidence for these units can be gained by direct observation of your work. You may be asked to provide the following types of evidence:

- Products. This might include a copy of progress notes or a care plan on mobility that you have completed. Remember to delete the resident's name to preserve confidentiality.
- Witness testimony. This is a statement from a senior member of staff. It might be a statement detailing how you have met certain performance criteria.
- Written work. You might be asked to prepare a piece of work about how you encourage residents to remain mobile. You might be asked to write a case history about a resident whom you have helped to remain mobile or become more mobile. You may be asked to discuss the difficulties you face in enabling people to move around the home and how you deal

with these difficulties. You might be asked to write an account of how you helped an individual prepare for a journey.

Your assessor will also use other methods to help you gain evidence for this unit. These may include:

- Verbal questioning
- Written questions

Simulations can be used to increase your awareness of mobility problems. One assessor borrowed wheelchairs and asked her students to spend the morning in town. Students soon found out how inaccessible many buildings are for wheelchair users. Others reported that they were ignored or treated differently because they were in wheelchairs. Students then began to realise why some older people dread leaving the home.

Simulations can also be used to assess your ability to meet performance criteria.

Chapter 10

Moving and Handling

Introduction

This chapter covers the option group A units Z7, Z7.1 and Z7.2 – 'contribute to the movement and handling of individuals to maximise their physical comfort'. Details on the option group unit Z7.3 – 'preventing and minimising the adverse effects of pressure' – are given in Chapter 11.

This chapter gives details of the legislation and policies relating to moving and handling. It outlines:

- Legal issues
- Employer responsibilities
- Employee responsibilities
- How great is the risk of back injury
- Patient handling policies
- Use of hoists and slings
- Training and education
- Information on moving and handling

Legal issues

The Health and Safety at Work Act 1974 outlined the responsibilities of employers to provide a safe working environment for staff. The Manual Handling Operations Regulations of 1992 became law on 1 January 1993. They aim to prevent back and other injury by making sure manual handling tasks are evaluated and reducing or eliminating the need for manual handling, wherever possible. Employers have legal duties to:

- So far as is reasonably practical, avoid the need for employees to undertake any manual handling operations at work which involve the risk of their being injured
- Undertake an adequate risk assessment for those tasks that cannot reasonably and practicably be avoided. Figure 10.1 illustrates the risk assessment process.

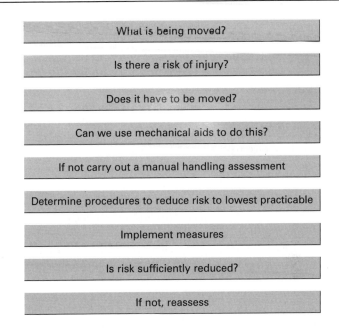

Fig. 10.1   Guide to manual handling responsibilities.

Manual handling regulations

All manual handling operations must be assessed. This means not only moving residents but also moving stores, laundry bags and other items. The Health and Safety Executive and the Health and Safety Commission have produced guidance to help reduce risks.

Every individual who requires manual handling should be assessed. The assessment should include the person's weight, factors affecting handling and methods to be used and equipment required to assist the person to move. This assessment should be recorded and kept with the resident's records.

The employer should also carry out risk assessments to reduce the risk of injury when lifting or moving everyday items such as the boxes of books received from the library, soap powder and supplies. The assessment should include the weight of such items and where they are to be stored.

Responsibilities of the employer

Employers are now obliged to take the following steps to reduce the incidence of back injury among staff:

- Eliminate manual handling wherever possible
- Assess all manual handling tasks

- Reduce the risk of injury where there is no alternative to lifting
- Ensure that staff are physically capable of carrying out their duties – pregnant staff and staff who have had a baby within the last three months should be assessed separately from other staff
- Ensure that all staff receive regular and appropriate training in moving and handling. This is normally part of the induction process. Ongoing training is incorporated within the home's training plan. Many homes employ staff who have received special training in moving and handling and are qualified to train staff. Sometimes smaller homes employ specially qualified trainers to carry out training sessions.
- Ensure that appropriate equipment is provided, maintained and monitored
- Monitor and record all accidents and sickness – take action to prevent accidents recurring wherever possible

Pregnant staff

Staff who are pregnant are less capable of lifting objects and more at risk during any manual handling procedures. In pregnancy, the ligaments supporting the spine loosen and the pregnant member of staff is at greater risk of back injury than any other member of staff. Most homes forbid pregnant staff to lift everyday items such as stores or to manually move residents under any circumstances. This means that the pregnant member of staff does not lift boxes of dressing packs, stationery or any equipment, and does not lift a patient even in an emergency. Some homes prohibit pregnant staff from taking any part in manual handling. In a small home the employer may consider that it is not possible to have a member of staff on duty who is not able to take part in manual handling. If, for example, there are only two staff on duty and one of them is unable to assist residents to move this would be unsafe. In these circumstances, the employer has a duty to find alternative work (at the same rate of pay) for the pregnant employee.

The employee has a duty to inform the employer as soon as she is aware of her pregnancy, so that steps can be taken to reduce the possible risk of injury to the member of staff, to other staff members and to residents.

The Health and Safety Executive

If it is 'reasonably practical' for the employer to meet legal requirements and the employer fails to do so, the Health and

Safety Executive can take action. Many residents enjoy showers but others prefer to bath. If a hoist is required to help heavily dependent residents bath but the employer fails to provide one, the Health and Safety Executive could intervene. The Health and Safety Executive employs health and safety inspectors who visit and assess risks. The older person and staff would be at risk of injury if they attempted to lift the individual in and out of the bath. In such circumstances the Health and Safety Executive would serve a notice obliging the employer to supply equipment. The inspector specifies a period of time in which the employer must comply. The inspector will then return to ensure that the equipment has been supplied. If the employer fails to comply, he or she may be prosecuted under the Health and Safety at Work Act 1974. Employers who fail to comply can be imprisoned for up to two years and face unlimited fines.

Lifting in emergencies

The Royal College of Nursing (RCN), a trade union and professional body for registered nurses, has been pressing for a no lifting policy for some years. Until 1993, it was considered acceptable for two nurses to lift patients weighing eight stone or less. In 1998, *The Guide to The Handling of Patients*, produced by the National Back Pain Association and the RCN, updated their guidance on manual handling. The latest guidance states that staff should not lift other than in an emergency. The emergencies identified are when the person is:

- In danger of drowning
- In an area that is on fire and filling with smoke
- In danger from bullet or bomb
- In danger from a collapsing building or other structure

This is guidance not law and does not ban lifting. However it may be used in the courts and referred to as 'best practice'.

Employee responsibilities

Employees have a duty under the legislation to take reasonable care of their own health and safety and those who may be affected by their omissions, and to co-operate with the employer. This means that employees:

- Have a duty to attend training sessions
- Should comply with moving and handling policies within the home

- Should not use manoeuvres designated as poor practice
- Should use equipment provided
- Should report any faults in equipment promptly
- Should remove dangerous equipment from use
- Should inform the employer of any risks identified
- Should inform the employer of any health problems that affect their ability to carry out their role.

How great is the risk of back injury?

Legislation states that employers should, so far as reasonably practical, avoid the need for employees to undertake any manual handling operations at work which involve the risk of their being injured.

But will it really hurt to lift a resident? The research suggests that staff working with older people are very much at risk of developing back pain and more likely to suffer injury as a result of lifting. One survey discovered that 28% of nurses working on surgical wards in NHS hospitals suffered from back pain at least once a week. In elderly care wards 92% of staff suffered from regular backpain. Research has shown that before the use of hoists became widespread an elderly care nurse could lift a ton during a shift. Moving and handling regulations aim to make this a thing of the past.

Backs can be injured not only by lifting or by accidents; they can also be injured by the strain of lifting day in and day out for years. Repetitive movements, poor posture, prolonged stooping, awkward postures and sudden movements can also cause back injury and pain.

Uniforms can increase the risk of back injury. In the UK, many female nursing staff no longer wear traditional dresses with narrow skirts. These are restrictive and make it more difficult to move freely. In other countries such as the United States and Australia research has shown that nurses who wear tunics and trousers are much less likely to suffer from back injury (Fig. 10.2). Increasingly British nurses are adopting practical uniforms to enable them to move easily and avoid the risk of injury.

Staff working with elderly people can, with the best of intentions, move and handle older people who with aids, instruction and encouragement could move themselves. This practice causes the older person to become more dependent on staff, reduces quality of life and increases staff workload. It is worth spending time encouraging and enabling an individual to move unassisted or with minimal help.

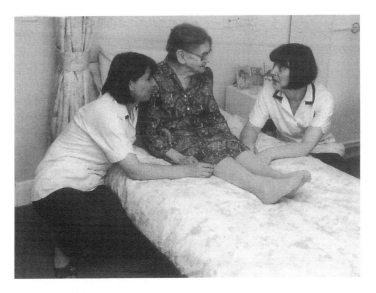

Fig. 10.2 Uniforms such as these reduce the risk of back injury because movement is unrestricted.

Moving and handling policies

Any resident who requires help to move should have a moving and handling assessment. It is good practice to complete a short assessment even on patients who do not require assistance. The assessment should indicate when the person requires help, what help is required and detail any aids that will be used. This assessment should be documented and referred to in the care plan. The assessment should be updated every six months, or sooner if the individual's needs change.

Many homes now have printed risk assessment forms. This form should be simple and easy to fill in. The risk assessment should be carried out by a competent registered nurse. In residential homes the risk assessment will be carried out by either the manager or a competent member of staff. If staff in homes require further advice they can contact the community physiotherapist or a manual handling specialist.

Care plans

The information from the manual handling assessment is used to draw up a plan of care to which staff should refer before handling. The care plan should specify:

- The equipment required to move the person. This may be a sliding sheet, hoist, standing hoist, frame, monkey pole or other piece of equipment.
- The number of staff required to carry out the handling procedure.
- The handling procedure. The procedure for assisting a person transfer from bed to chair will differ from that used to help the person transfer from chair to toilet. The care plan should give details of each handling procedure, e.g. bathing, using the toilet or moving from wheelchair to armchair.
- How the person can help with the transfer.
- Any difficulties or constraints, e.g. the person may be confused and need reassurance and time to enable safe moving and handling.
- Any other information that staff require.

Care plans should be reviewed regularly. If the person's abilities change and the methods of handling change these must be noted on the care plan.

Training

The Guide to the Handling of Patients (revised 4th edition) states that all staff should receive training in moving and handling before being required to move people.

Employers have a legal duty to provide training to enable staff to move patients and to avoid injury. The latest recommendations are that all staff receive classroom-based training on induction. The training required will depend on the previous level of training but should be between two and five days. Training courses should include:

- The home's moving and handling policy
- Information about how the spine functions and how back pain is caused
- Principles of assessing risk and assessing the patient
- Assessing risk and assessing the patient
- How to teach the patient to move unaided
- The environment and equipment – known as ergonomics
- Handling aids
- Manual handling techniques
- General health awareness including awareness of good movement at work and at home
- Responsibilities for reporting risks and injuries

Training and supervision should continue in the home. Staff should receive regular refresher courses. The current recommendation is that all staff should receive a minimum of one day a year; this can either be workplace or classroom-based.

Training records

Employers now keep records of training as they may be needed for legal reasons. When you complete a training course your employer may ask you to sign a form stating that you have attended the course and are aware of the home's policies relating to moving and handling and assessment.

Equipment

The employer is required to provide a range of appropriate equipment to enable staff to handle safely patients and loads such as soap powder, kitchen stores etc. In a nursing home the range of equipment available to move residents may include hoists, standing hoists, transfer boards, handling belts, monkey poles and sliding sheets. Residential homes caring for people who are unable to move unaided must provide appropriate equipment to enable the individual to be moved safely. Increasingly insurers demand evidence of risk assessment and details of staff training and equipment provided before agreeing to insure the home.

Using hoists and slings

Despite the fact that employers provide hoists and have introduced no lifting or safer lifting policies, staff continue to lift patients manually, risking the health of the patient, their own health and that of their colleagues. Research shows that there are a number of reasons why staff do not use hoists, including:

- Insufficient room to move the hoist around
- The hoist will not fit in the toilet or bathroom
- The hoist is poorly maintained – the wheels may stick or staff may struggle to use it
- Staff have not been trained to use the hoist
- The resident (or relatives) do not like the hoist and do not understand why staff insist on using it
- Other staff do not use the hoist

Staff education and training enable staff to learn how to use equipment and the home's policies and procedures ensure that problems with equipment and space are reported so that action can be taken.

Hoists are used to move people. There are a number of different hoists on the market. Figures 10.3, 10.4 and 10.5 show some examples. If the home is considering buying a new hoist a representative from the company will show staff how to use the hoist. Staff are trained to use new hoists and an instruction booklet is supplied so that staff can refer to it. The patient is held in a sling or a seat that is attached to the hoist. There are different types of slings and these are used for different purposes. Two piece slings with one part placed behind the patient's back and another placed under the thighs should no longer be used with elderly people. The Department of Health has instructed homes caring for older people not to use these slings because serious accidents have occurred.

Figure 10.6 shows a selection of slings.

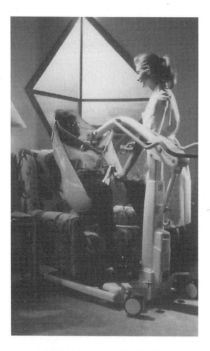

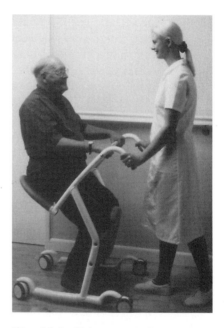

Fig. 10.3 Using a Trixie hoist to move a resident from a chair.

Fig. 10.4 Using a standing hoist to help a person stand.

Preparing for moving and handling

It is important to make sure that you have enough space to move. Move equipment and furniture if necessary. If the person requires help to move you may find it easier to rearrange the furniture in the room. If the bed is against the wall and two staff are required to

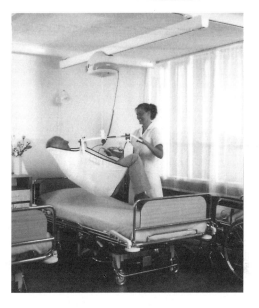

Fig. 10.5 An overhead hoist is unobtrusive and space saving.

help move the person it makes sense to rearrange the furniture so that staff have access to both sides of the bed. Remember though that this is the person's home; obtain consent before moving furniture. If the person wants the bed in a particular position you may have to move the bed out to ensure access each time you help the person to move.

Avoid moving people who can move independently. The person is at risk of becoming physically weaker and losing the ability to move independently. Ensure that you have enough people and the correct equipment to move the person. Explain what you intend to do. Ask the person to co-operate. Explain what you wish the person to do and check that the person has understood.

Turning a person in bed

People who are unable to turn over in bed without help are at risk of developing pressure sores. Details on preventing pressure sores are given in Chapter 11. If the person is unable to turn over unaided you must turn the person. A range of equipment is available to enable you to slide and turn the patient.

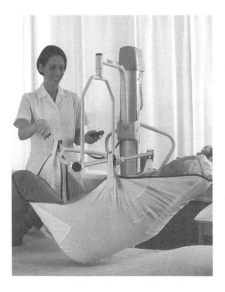 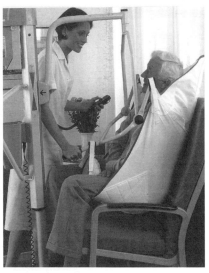

Using a manual hoist to help a resident get up.

Positioning a person in a chair using a battery powered hoist.

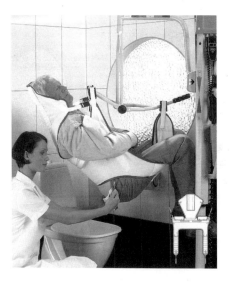

A hoist and toileting sling enable the person's clothing to be adjusted easily when helping them to use the toilet.

Fig. 10.6   A selection of slings.

Educating staff and promoting safe practice

According to a report by a clinical standards advisory group in 1994, back pain cost the NHS £480 million a year. Although the moving and handling regulations were introduced in 1993, a study commissioned by the Royal College of Nursing in 1996 showed that the level of back injury had not fallen. The RCN believe that this is because more patients are now cared for in community settings. At the time of writing they plan a research project to check how nursing homes are fulfilling their legal responsibilities. But only 25% of all nurses work in the independent sector. If policies were being effectively implemented in NHS hospitals, surely the injury rate would be falling. Research indicates that only half of all NHS hospitals comply with their legislative duties. Even then, we would expect the injury rate to fall in the hospitals that complied. Managers in all settings are aware of hoists and equipment left to gather dust as staff carry on lifting patients. We need to educate staff and reinforce good practice. We need to stop moving people around so much and encourage those who can move to move themselves.

Summary

Ten years ago many nursing staff lifted people without considering how this practice could injure patients and staff. Now things are different. Before we move people or objects we must consider the safest and most sensible way to do this. Ten years ago there were few aids to enable us to move people; now we have a large range of equipment and aids to enable us to move patients safely and to avoid risk of staff injury. Modern moving and handling techniques aim to encourage people, wherever possible, to move independently using aids and equipment when required. Modern techniques aim to avoid injury to patients and staff and to make homes and hospitals safer places for those who provide care and those who require it.

Portfolio preparation

Your assessor must have evidence that you can meet the performance criteria for this unit. Before beginning this unit discuss assessment strategies with your assessor. Most of the evidence for this unit can be gained by direct observation of your work. You may be asked to provide the following types of evidence:

- Products. This might include watching you assist a resident to get into bed or get up. This might be supplemented by questioning about the care plan and the reasons for using certain methods to assist the individual, and more general questions about moving and handling.
- Witness testimony. This is a statement from a senior member of staff. It might detail how you have met certain assessment criteria.
- Written work. You might be asked to write an account of how you helped a particular resident to move and the aids and techniques used.

Your assessor may also use other methods to help you gain evidence for this unit. These may include:

- Verbal questioning
- Written questions

Simulations can be used to assess your ability to use equipment for moving and handling

Further information

You may be able to find these publications in your college library or your manager may have copies.

Health and Safety Executive (1992) *Management of Health and Safety at Work*. Stationery Office, London.

Health and Safety Executive (1998) *Management of Health and Safety at Work*. Stationery Office, London.

Health and Safety Executive (1992) *Manual Handling Guidance on Regulations*. Stationery Office, London.

Health and Safety Commission (1992) *Management of Health and Safety at Work*. Approved Code of Practice. Stationery Office, London.

Management of Health and Safety at Work Regulations (1992) *Statutory Instrument no. 2051*. Stationery Office, London.

Further reading

National Back Pain Association and Royal College of Nursing (1998) *The Guide to the Handling of Patients. Introducing a safer handling policy*, revised 4th edition. National Back Pain Association and Royal College of Nursing, Teddington, Middlesex.

Chapter 11

Preventing Pressure Sores

Introduction

This chapter provides information on the option group A unit Z7.3 – 'assist individuals to prevent and minimise the adverse effects of pressure'.

This chapter provides information on:

- How pressure sores develop
- Treating pressure sores
- Where pressure sores develop
- Which individuals are most at risk and why
- Assessing risk
- The principles of preventing pressure sores
- Using aids such as beds, mattresses, cushions, heel and elbow protectors
- Caring for the whole person

Pressure sores

Pressure sores are commonly called bedsores. Doctors and nurses often refer to them by the technical name of decubitus ulcers. They will be referred to throughout this chapter as pressure sores.

Pressure sores are caused by pressure, friction or shearing forces applied to the skin. A person does not have to be confined to bed to develop pressure sores. Many people who are sitting in chairs all day are in danger of developing pressure sores. Pressure sores are areas of skin that have been damaged by unrelieved pressure, friction or shearing forces or a combination of these three factors.

How pressure sores develop

Pressure sores develop when a part of the body is not moved. Normally the skin is nourished by small blood vessels called capillaries. Capillaries carry blood that delivers oxygen and glucose to the skin. If blood supply to the skin is cut off, the skin and deeper tissues die. Unrelieved pressure on any area of the body interrupts the capillary blood flow and can lead to tissue death. Poor moving and handling techniques, which drag rather than lift, are known as shearing forces. This can cause tissue damage that leads to the development of pressure sores.

Normally when a person begins to develop a pressure sore, the first sign is a red mark on the skin. If you place a finger lightly on the red area and it whitens, this shows that the capillary circulation is undamaged. If you act quickly, you may be able to help prevent a pressure sore developing. If the skin remains red when light finger pressure is applied, capillary circulation has been damaged. There may be a slight sore or blister on the skin. It will worsen if you do not act promptly and seek advice.

At one time, it was recommended that reddened skin was massaged. It was thought that a firm massage improved the circulation and got the blood flowing back into the reddened skin. However, researchers found that massaging reddened skin did not improve circulation and actually caused further damage and made it more likely that the person would develop pressure sores. Reddened skin should not under any circumstances be massaged.

Pressure sore grading

If action is not taken to relieve pressure regularly, areas of reddened skin can quickly develop into serious pressure sores. There are five stages of pressure sores:

(1) One or more red areas of skin that whiten when you press a finger lightly on the skin
(2) One or more red areas of skin that remain red when you press a finger lightly on the skin
(3) Ulcer visible on skin
(4) Skin and fat beneath the skin is ulcerated and muscle underneath is swollen
(5) Skin, fat, muscle and sometimes bone damaged by pressure

Pressure sore sites

Pressure sores can develop on any part of the body (Fig. 11.1). They can occur on ears, cheeks, arms, trunk, legs and heels. Most pressure sores develop between the buttocks on the bony area known as the sacrum. Anyone who is unable to move and who is

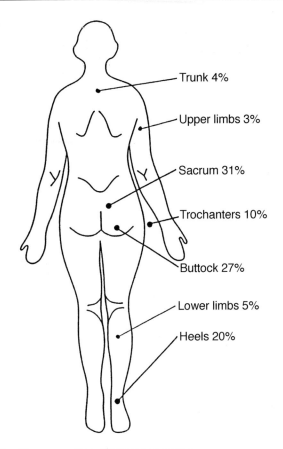

Trunk 4%

Upper limbs 3%

Sacrum 31%

Trochanters 10%

Buttock 27%

Lower limbs 5%

Heels 20%

Fig. 11.1   Common sites of pressure sores.

not helped to move can develop a pressure sore after a few hours. Pressure sores are not caused by bedrest; people sitting in chairs also develop sacral pressure sores.

The heels are also a common site for pressure sores. A person sitting with heels resting on a footstool is just as much at risk as the person whose heels are resting on a mattress in bed.

Who is at risk of developing pressure sores?

Older people are 20 times more likely to develop pressure sores than people in their twenties and thirties. Women are more likely to develop pressure sores than men, because women have a higher proportion of body fat than men. Fat has poorer blood supply than muscle or lean tissue. People who suffer from a long-standing illness are more likely to develop pressure sores than people in good health. Most older people living in homes have been admitted because of poor health and therefore are at greater risk of developing pressure sores than people who live in their own homes. Some older people are at greater risk than others.

Confused people

People who are confused are at risk of developing pressure sores. Normally if we are forced to sit still for a long time, perhaps on a car journey, we unconsciously adjust our weight to reduce the effects of pressure. People who are confused are often unable to work out the cause of discomfort and adjust position. Many people who are confused sit quietly for hours and staff may be busy attending to more alert people who are able to ask for help. The confused person may not be aware of the discomfort or pain caused by remaining in one position for a long time. Sometimes the person is aware of the discomfort but is unable to explain. Sometimes people who are confused are prescribed sedatives. This may be because the person is agitated or wanders around. Sedatives can cause more problems than they solve. Sedatives can make older people drowsy and less aware. People who are drowsy will be less aware of pain and discomfort.

People who are unable to walk or move without help

Normally people who are able to move around will feel stiff and uncomfortable if they are sitting or lying in one position. Getting up and walking or rolling over in bed will relieve pressure and prevent tissue damage. People who are unable to move around without help rely on staff to help them turn over, get up or change position. If an older person at high risk of developing pressure sores is not moved or helped to move, severe skin damage can occur and a deep pressure sore can develop.

People who are paralysed

People who have suffered from strokes may be paralysed down one side of the body. The person may not be able to feel anything on the paralysed side and may be unaware of discomfort and pressure. The person may need help to get up or change position. Stroke can affect the ability to communicate. The person may be unable to let you know she is uncomfortable and needs help to move.

People who suffer from diseases of the brain (referred to as neurological diseases), such as multiple sclerosis or motor neurone disease, may lose all sensation in the lower part of the body. As the disease advances people may have difficulty in moving and speaking.

People with heart disease and high blood pressure

People with heart disease and high blood pressure are at risk of developing pressure sores because they have poor circulation. When circulation is poor skin becomes more sensitive to the effects of pressure and is more easily damaged.

People with diabetes

Diabetes becomes more common as people age. Approximately 10% of 85 year olds have diabetes. People from some ethnic backgrounds are more likely to develop diabetes. Approximately 14% of older people from Afro-Caribbean backgrounds develop diabetes; and 20% of people of Indian or Pakistani descent develop diabetes in old age. People with diabetes often suffer from poor circulation. People who have mild diabetes, which is treated with a special diet, are less at risk than diabetics who require tablets to help control diabetes. People who require insulin injections to control diabetes are more likely to suffer from poor circulation than other diabetics.

Some people with diabetes, especially those, who require insulin injections, develop loss of feeling in the feet, lower parts of the legs and the hands. This condition is known as peripheral neuropathy, and there is no treatment for it. People with diabetes are at great risk of developing pressure sores on the heels, as they are often unaware of pain or discomfort caused by pressure. Poor circulation and the effects of diabetes, which slow down the rate of wound healing, make it difficult to heal such pressure sores if they develop.

People who are overweight or underweight

People who are overweight or underweight are more likely to develop pressure sores. Overweight people have poorer circulation than people of normal weight. Many overweight people have a poor diet that is too high in sugars and low in vitamins. A diet low in vitamins affects the health of the skin and increases the risk of pressure sores.

Underweight people are even more likely than overweight people to develop pressure sores. Thin people lack a layer of fat that protects muscle from the effects of pressure, and thin people are much more at risk of the effects of shearing forces because their bones are more prominent.

People who are incontinent

People who are incontinent of faeces and urine are at greater risk of developing pressure sores than those who are incontinent of urine only. People who are incontinent can develop skin rashes if pads are not changed frequently or if the skin is not carefully washed after each episode of incontinence. Urine, especially concentrated urine, can burn the skin. People who are incontinent of faeces may wet on a soiled pad. This causes the release of ammonia and can cause skin to become sore and red very quickly. Skin soreness and rashes cause the skin to become inflamed. Sore, inflamed skin can develop blisters and boils. These can become infected. People who have sore or infected skin are more at risk of developing pressure sores than people who have healthy skin.

Many people who are incontinent wear pads. If pads are not put on properly, ridges from the pad can cause pressure on the skin and this can lead to pressure sores. There are many different types of pad. The quality of pad varies, as does the cost. All pads are made of paper (cellulose) pulp. This is covered by a one way liner that is designed to draw urine away from the patient's skin and into the pad. Most pads have a plastic backing to prevent urine leaking onto the patient's clothes. Some pads contain more pulp than others. Some pads also contain super absorbent crystals. The crystals turn into a gel and lock urine into the pad. Good quality pads draw urine away from the skin quickly and keep the skin drier between changes. Skin that is not soaked in urine is less likely to become sore, infected or develop pressure sores.

The effects of pressure sores

Pressure sores can cause a great deal of pain and discomfort. If the person develops a pressure sore on a heel it can make walking difficult and painful and can prevent the person walking. Pain can prevent an older person moving around, chatting and taking part in the activities of the home. Pain can prevent the older person from getting a good night's sleep. Doctors can prescribe painkillers, and people with large or deep pressure sores may require strong painkillers. Unfortunately strong painkillers can make some people feel sick and can cause constipation. Lack of sleep can make the individual feel unwell.

Pressure sores, especially those on the sacrum and the hips, can easily become infected. Infection can cause the person to develop a high temperature and to feel unwell. The individual may feel too unwell to eat, yet a diet full of protein, vitamins and carbohydrates is essential if the wound is to heal.

People who have infected wounds are usually prescribed antibiotics by their doctors. Antibiotics can make some people feel sick and lose their appetites. Some people can also suffer from diarrhoea when prescribed antibiotics.

Infected wounds often smell. Some wounds, because of the bacteria with which they are infected, smell dreadful. This can be very upsetting for the patient. Some people who develop deep pressure sores can suffer from infection that infects the bone. They can develop blood poisoning (septicaemia) and even with hospital treatment, some people will not survive.

People who have developed pressure sores will require wound dressings. These will be carried out by registered nurses in nursing homes; in residential homes, the district nurse will visit to carry out dressings. Many older people who have developed pressure sores become depressed. Some are so depressed that they feel life is not worth living and require antidepressant tablets.

How registered nurses discover who is at risk of developing pressure sores

Care assistants in nursing homes work with registered nurses (RNs). Often you will be responsible for caring for a small group of residents, although of course you will help care for everyone within the home. The RN works with residents and staff to plan, manage, and deliver care. RNs use assessment tools to find out which residents are most at risk of developing pressure sores and how great the risk is. The nurse can then plan care to prevent pressure sores developing. Preventing pressure sores is a team effort and your role in preventing pressure sores is an important one.

There are over a dozen scales to assess the risk of developing pressure sores. The Norton scale and the Waterlow scale are the most popular but the Braden scale is becoming more widely used. The Norton scale (Fig. 11.2) was developed in 1962. It assesses the patient's general health, mental state, activity, mobility and continence. People score points based on these categories. An individual in poor health, who is confused, immobile and incontinent, will have a lower score than an individual who is in poor health but who is alert, walks with help and is continent. The total points are added up and this is known as the Norton score. A

Physical condition		Mental state		Activity		Mobility		Incontinence	
Good	4	Alert	4	Ambulant	4	Full	4	None	4
Fair	3	Apathetic	3	Walks with		Slightly		Occasional	3
Poor	2	Confused	2	help	3	limited	3	Usually	
Very bad	1	Stuporous	1	Chairbound	2	Very		urinary	2
				Bedfast	1	limited	2	Double	1
						Immobile	1		

Patient total score:
Implications:

Fig. 11.2   The Norton scale.

score of 16 points or below indicates that the person is at risk of developing a pressure sore. The lower the score the higher the risk of the person developing pressure sores.

The Waterlow scale (Fig. 11.3) was developed as a result of research carried out in 1985, and is a more detailed assessment scale. It assesses factors such as build, weight, continence, skin type, mobility, sex, age and appetite. The score has special high risk factors such as surgery, medication, age and diseases. Each risk factor carries points and the points are added up. A score of 10 indicates that the person is at risk of developing pressure sores; a score of 15–20 indicates that the person is at high risk; and a score of more than 20 indicates that the person is at very high risk. The higher the score the greater the risk of the person developing pressure sores.

The Braden Scale (Fig. 11.4) was developed in America in 1992. Many nurses caring for older people consider it more accurate than the other scores. The individual's condition is assessed using six very specific categories. The maximum score is twenty and the minimum is five. Anyone with a score of sixteen or less is considered at risk of developing a pressure sore. The lower the score the higher the risk.

Using an assessment tool enables RNs to identify people who are at high risk and to plan care that will prevent pressure sores developing. People admitted to nursing homes normally have a pressure sore risk assessment completed when they enter the home. People living in residential homes used to be more able, more mobile and less at risk of developing pressure sores. However, research suggests that very frail older people are now being admitted to residential homes. People entering residential homes do not normally have a pressure sore risk assessment carried out on admission. If you work in a residential home and are caring for people who are at risk of developing pressure sores, observe their skin carefully. If you think an individual's skin is deteriorating,

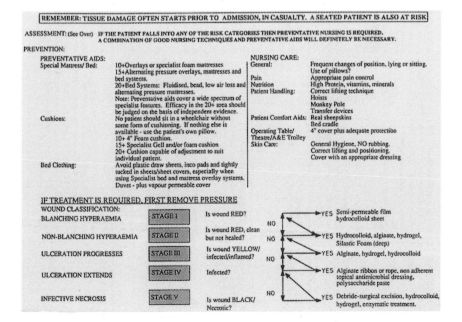

WATERLOW PRESSURE SORE PREVENTION/TREATMENT POLICY

RING SCORES IN TABLE, ADD TOTAL. SEVERAL SCORES PER CATEGORY CAN BE USED

BUILD/WEIGHT FOR HEIGHT	★	SKIN TYPE VISUAL RISK AREAS	★	SEX AGE	★	SPECIAL RISKS	★
AVERAGE	0	HEALTHY	0	MALE	1	TISSUE MALNUTRITION	★
ABOVE AVERAGE	1	TISSUE PAPER	1	FEMALE	2		
OBESE	2	DRY	1	14 - 49	1	e.g.: TERMINAL CACHEXIA	8
BELOW AVERAGE	3	OEDEMATOUS	1	50 - 64	2	CARDIAC FAILURE	5
		CLAMMY (TEMP↑)	1	65 - 74	3	PERIPHERAL VASCULAR	
CONTINENCE	★	DISCOLOURED	2	75 - 80	4	DISEASE	5
		BROKEN/SPOT	3	81+	5	ANAEMIA	2
COMPLETE/						SMOKING	1
CATHETERISED	0	MOBILITY	★	APPETITE	★	NEUROLOGICAL DEFICIT	★
OCCASION INCONT	1						
CATH/INCONTINENT							
OF FAECES	2	FULLY	0	AVERAGE	0	eg: DIABETES, M.S, CVA,	
DOUBLY INCONT	3	RESTLESS/FIDGETY	1	POOR	1	MOTOR/SENSORY	
		APATHETIC	2	N.G. TUBE/		PARAPLEGIA	4 - 6
		RESTRICTED	3	FLUIDS ONLY	2		
		INERT/TRACTION	4	NBM/ANOREXIC	3	MAJOR SURGERY/TRAUMA	★
		CHAIRBOUND	5				
						ORTHOPAEDIC -	
						BELOW WAIST,SPINAL	5
						ON TABLE > 2 HOURS	5
SCORE	10+ AT RISK	15+ HIGH RISK	20+ VERY HIGH RISK			MEDICATION	★
						CYTOTOXICS,	4
						HIGH DOSE STEROIDS	
						ANTI-INFLAMMATORY	

© J Waterlow 1991 Revised March 1992

OBTAINABLE FROM: NEWTONS, CURLAND, TAUNTON, TA3 5SG

REMEMBER: TISSUE DAMAGE OFTEN STARTS PRIOR TO ADMISSION, IN CASUALTY. A SEATED PATIENT IS ALSO AT RISK

ASSESSMENT: (See Over) IF THE PATIENT FALLS INTO ANY OF THE RISK CATEGORIES THEN PREVENTATIVE NURSING IS REQUIRED.
A COMBINATION OF GOOD NURSING TECHNIQUES AND PREVENTATIVE AIDS WILL DEFINITELY BE NECESSARY.

PREVENTION:

PREVENTATIVE AIDS:
Special Mattress/ Bed: 10+Overlays or specialist foam mattresses
15+Alternating pressure overlays, mattresses and bed systems.
20+Bed Systems: Fluidised, bead, low air loss and alternating pressure mattresses.
Note: Preventative aids cover a wide spectrum of specialist features. Efficacy in the 20+ area should be judged on the basis of independent evidence.

Cushions: No patient should sit in a wheelchair without some form of cushioning. If nothing else is available - use the patient's own pillow.
10+ 4" Foam cushion.
15+ Specialist Gell and/or foam cushion
20+ Cushion capable of adjustment to suit individual patient.

Bed Clothing: Avoid plastic draw sheets, inco pads and tightly tucked in sheets/sheet covers, especially when using Specialist bed and mattress overlay systems.
Duvet - plus vapour permeable cover

NURSING CARE:
General: Frequent changes of position, lying or sitting.
Use of pillows?
Pain Appropriate pain control
Nutrition High Protein, vitamins, minerals
Patient Handling: Correct lifting technique
Hoists
Monkey Pole
Transfer devices
Patient Comfort Aids: Real sheepskins
Bed cradle
Operating Table/ 4" cover plus adequate protection
Theatre/A&E Trolley
Skin Care: General Hygiene, NO rubbing.
Correct lifting and positioning.
Cover with an appropriate dressing.

IF TREATMENT IS REQUIRED, FIRST REMOVE PRESSURE

WOUND CLASSIFICATION:

BLANCHING HYPERAEMIA	STAGE I	Is wound RED?	YES Semi-permeable film hydrocolloid sheet
NON-BLANCHING HYPERAEMIA	STAGE II	Is wound RED, clean but not healed?	YES Hydrocolloid, alginate, hydrogel, Silastic Foam (deep)
ULCERATION PROGRESSES	STAGE III	Is wound YELLOW/ infected/inflamed?	YES Alginate, hydrogel, hydrocolloid
ULCERATION EXTENDS	STAGE IV	Infected?	YES Alginate ribbon or rope, non adherent topical antimicrobial dressing, polysaccharide paste
INFECTIVE NECROSIS	STAGE V	Is wound BLACK/ Necrotic?	YES Debride-surgical excision, hydrocolloid, hydrogel, enzymatic treatment.

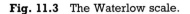

Fig. 11.3 The Waterlow scale.

BRADEN SCALE

	1	2	3	4
SENSORY PERCEPTION ability to respond meaningfully to pressure-related discomfort	**1. Completely Limited** Unresponsive (does not moan, flinch, or grasp) to painful stimuli, due to diminished level of consciousness or sedation OR limited ability to feel pain over most body surfaces	**2. Very Limited** Responds only to painful stimuli. Cannot communicate discomfort except by moaning or restlessness OR Has a sensory impairment which limits the ability to feel pain or discomfort over 1/2 of body	**3. Slightly Limited** Responds to verbal commands but cannot always communicate discomfort or need to be turned OR Has some sensory impairment which limits ability to feel pain or discomfort in 1 or 2 extremities	**4. No Impairment** Responds to verbal commands. Has no sensory deficit which would affect ability to feel or voice pain or discomfort
MOISTURE degree to which skin is exposed to moisture	**1. Constantly Moist** Skin is kept moist almost constantly by perspiration, urine, etc. Dampness is detected every time patient is moved or turned.	**2. Very Moist** Skin is often, but not always moist. Linen must be changed at least once a shift.	**3. Occasionally Moist** Skin is occasionally moist, requiring an extra linen change approximately once a day	**4. Rarely Moist** Skin is usually dry. Linen only requires changing at routine intervals
ACTIVITY degree of physical activity	**. Bedfast** Confined to bed	**2. Chairfast** Ability to walk severely limited or non-existent. Cannot bear own weight and/or must be assisted into chair or wheelchair	**3. Walks Occasionally** Walks occasionally during day, but for very short distances, with or without assistance. Spends majority of each shift in bed or chair	**4. Walks Frequently** Walks outside the room at least twice a day and inside room at least once every 2 hours during walking hours
MOBILITY ability to change and control body position	**1. Completely Immobile** Does not make even slight changes in body or extremity position without assistance	**2. Very Limited** Makes occasional slight changes in body or extremity position but unable to make frequent or significant changes independently	**3. Slightly Limited** Makes frequent though slight changes in body or extremity position independently	**4. No Limitation** Makes major and frequent changes in position without assistance
NUTRITION usual food intake pattern	**1. Very Poor** Never eats a complete meal. Rarely eats more than 1/3 of any food offered. Eats 2 servings or less of protein (meat or dairy products) per day. Fluids taken poorly. Does not take a liquid dietary supplement OR is NBM and/or maintained on clear liquids or IV's for more than 5 days	**2. Probably Inadequate** Rarely eats a complete meal and generally eats only 1/2 of any food offered. Protein intake includes only 3 servings of meat or dairy products per day. Occasionally will take a dietary supplement OR Receives less than optimum amount of liquid diet or tube feeding	**3. Adequate** Eats over half of most meals. Eats a total of 4 servings of protein (meat, dairy products) each day. Occasionally will refuse a meal, but will usually take a supplement if offered OR is on a tube feeding or TPN regimen which probably meets most of nutritional needs	**4. Excellent** Eats most of every meal Never refuses a meal Usually eats a total 4 or more servings of meat and dairy products Occasionally eats between meals. Does not require supplementation
FRICTION AND SHEAR	**1. Problem** Requires moderate to maximum assistance in moving. Complete lifting without sliding against sheets is impossible. Frequently slides down in bed or chair, requiring frequent repositioning with maximum assistance. Spasticity, contractures or agitation leads to almost constant friction.	**2. Potential Problem** Moves freely or requires minimum assistance. During a move skin probably slides to some extent against sheets, chair restraints or other devices. Maintains relatively good position in chair or bed most of the time but occasionally slides down.	**3. No Apparent Problem** Moves in bed and in chair independently and has sufficient muscle strength to lift up completely during move. Maintains good position in bed or chair at all times.	

Fig. 11.4 The Braden scale.

inform your manager or a senior member of staff at once. The district nurse will normally be called and asked to carry out an assessment.

People living in residential homes who are at very high risk of developing a pressure sore may require nursing home care. Residential homes must abide by the legislation. This states that people living in residential homes should receive the care that could be given at home by a caring relative. The older person at high risk of developing a pressure sore will require higher levels of care than most residential homes can provide. This is because residential homes do not have the resources, facilities or aids that can be provided in nursing homes.

When a pressure sore risk assessment has been carried out in a nursing home, the RN will file a copy in the care plan. This will give the date of the assessment and details of the scale used. If the score indicates that the person is at risk, a plan of care will be written. This will explain how the team will work to prevent pressure sores occurring.

In residential homes, the district nurse will leave details of care in the person's case notes. These are left in the home so that other district nurses who call are aware of treatment required. The district nurse will leave instructions on how to prevent pressure sores and the care assistant caring for the person, or the manager, should record these instructions.

Preventing pressure sores

Most pressure sores can be prevented. The development of a pressure sore, in most cases, is a sign that care is not of a high standard and that staff failed to take action to prevent the sore developing. Staff who understand why pressure sores develop can act to prevent them occurring. Pressure sores are caused by unrelieved pressure that affects blood flow and causes sores to develop. Relieving the pressure and moving people allows blood to flow normally to the tissues and prevents pressure sores developing. People who are sitting in a chair all day are just as much at risk of developing pressure sores as people who are nursed in bed.

People who are sitting in chairs and who are able to walk should be encouraged to do so. Encouraging and helping an older person to walk to the dining room for lunch will help prevent a pressure sore. Serving lunch on a tray may mean the individual continues to sit and pressure on the bottom is unrelieved.

Many people need help and encouragement to walk. You should encourage residents to walk, walking with them and encouraging them to walk at their own pace. Offering to wheel a person, who is capable of walking, to the dining area does little to relieve pressure and help circulation. People who are unable to walk can be encouraged to stand. The person can use a Zimmer frame, grab rails or standing hoist or be helped by staff. Encouraging people to stand, even with help, not only helps prevent pressure sores but also prevents joints becoming stiff and reduces the risk of the patient's legs developing deformities such as flexion contractures. Details of flexion contractures are given in Chapter 9. People who are unable to walk or stand are at risk of pressure sores and should not sit all day in the same chair, as this will almost certainly cause pressure sores.

Older people require less sleep than younger people do and tire more easily than when they were young. Older people are more likely to have a nap in the afternoon and often sleep for an hour after lunch. In some homes, older people fall asleep in their chairs after lunch. They may awake feeling stiff, uncomfortable and not refreshed by their sleep.

Encouraging frail older people who feel tired to go to bed for a nap will help prevent pressure sores. You can assist the individual to bed and can help the person to lie on one side, which will relieve pressure on the bottom. The older person will sleep comfortably and awake refreshed ready for a cup of tea, a visit from family or friends or activities in the home.

People normally turn over in bed while they are asleep. Moving around in bed prevents us from developing pressure sores while we sleep. Many frail older people who are at risk of pressure sores are unable to turn over in bed. All people who are at risk should be turned every two hours. The person is normally nursed on his back for two hours, then turned onto perhaps the left side. Two hours later the person is turned onto the right side. If a patient's sacrum is becoming red, they may lie on one hip and then the other, avoiding wherever possible any pressure on the sacrum. If one of the hips is becoming red, the person may lie only on the other hip or on the sacrum. If a person is lying on their side there is a risk that they will roll back onto their back. A soft pillow is often placed either under the mattress or at the back of the patient, to prevent this.

Mattresses and beds used to prevent pressure sores developing

Older people who are at risk of developing pressure sores may still develop pressure sores even if turned every two hours. It can be difficult to turn people more frequently. Often two staff are needed to turn the patient. If two staff work together the person is at less risk of shearing forces that can cause pressure sores, and care assistants reduce the risk of developing a back injury. Details on moving and handling people are given in Chapter 10.

People who are turned every hour have little opportunity to rest or sleep. Many different types of mattresses and mattress overlays have been designed to reduce the risk of pressure sores developing. Pressure relieving equipment usually either replaces the existing mattress or lies on top of the existing mattress.

Pressure relieving mattresses and overlays

These aim to relieve the pressure that can lead to pressure sores developing (Fig. 11.5). They are normally made of horizontal cells of air, which inflate and deflate on a cycle. This cycle is controlled by an electrical pump. The alternate cells that are inflated support the patient, while the deflated cells are relieving the pressure to that area of the patient's body. Alternating pressure mattresses/overlays are sometimes referred to as ripple mattresses. Pressure relieving mattresses are used for the prevention of pressure sores and also the treatment of any existing sores.

Some pressure relieving mattresses/overlays automatically adjust the amount of air in the cells. They are able to adjust to the weight and position of the individual. Others, however, have a small dial that needs to be set according to the weight of the

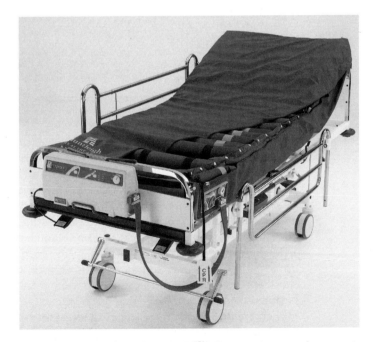

Fig. 11.5 Alternating pressure relieving mattress replacement.

patient. There is normally a printed table on the electronic pump giving details about which settings should be used for people within certain weight ranges.

Pressure relieving mattresses and overlays (Figs 11.6 and 11.7) are used for all levels of risk and grade of pressure sore. It is important that you seek advice from a registered nurse if you are unsure which product is suitable for an individual.

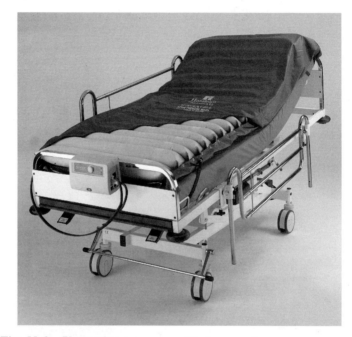

Fig. 11.6 Alternating pressure relieving overlay.

Some foam and fibre pressure relieving mattresses/overlays have a special vapour permeable multi-stretch cover. This vapour permeability allows the patient's skin to breathe and prevents the person from becoming hot and sweaty. This means that the skin is less likely to become macerated. The covers are water-resistant and the multi-stretch properties help to prevent the cover wrinkling and bunching up and reduce friction. Manufacturers recommend that the covers are washed with soap and water. Disinfectants, detergents and deodorisers should not be sprayed onto the covers. If you are unsure, ask your manager who will check the manufacturer's cleaning guidance.

When using a pressure relieving mattress/overlay, the sheet should not be tucked in tightly and Kylie-type bedsheets, draw sheets and incontinence pads should be kept to a minimum as they

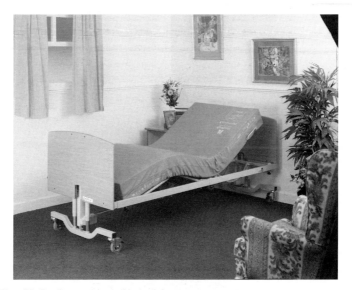

Fig. 11.7 Pressure reducing foam mattress.

may reduce the effectiveness of pressure relieving mattresses. It is best to leave the pressure relieving mattress/overlay switched on even when not in use. The motor has to work harder to re-inflate than to maintain the inflated pressure. Deflating the mattress means that the individual cannot go back to bed if tired, as the mattress/overlay should be inflated before the person uses it.

Some pressure reducing overlays and mattresses can also be made of foam or fibre. These reduce pressure by moulding to the contours of the body so that there is a greater surface area in contact with the overlay. This distributes the weight more evenly and reduces the pressure.

Pressure reducing overlays and mattresses should only be used to prevent pressure sores. They are not suitable for people who have developed pressure sores. These types of mattresses/overlays are normally used to help prevent pressure sores in people who are at low to medium risk of developing them. It is important to seek advice from a registered nurse who can check the manufacturer's recommendations. These mattresses and overlays are available with vapour permeable covers.

In some nursing homes, hospices and hospitals specialised beds such as low air loss (Fig. 11.8) and fluidised bead beds are sometimes used for people who are very ill, have existing pressure sores and cannot easily be moved. If you require any further information on these specialised beds, ask a registered nurse or obtain details from the manufacturers (details are given at the end of the chapter).

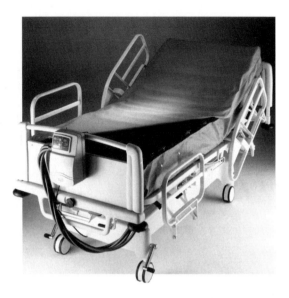

Fig. 11.8   Low airloss mattress replacement.

Cushions and pressure relieving aids

People who are at risk of developing pressure sores are at even greater risk when they are sitting in chairs. A range of cushions should be available within the home to help prevent and treat pressure sores. In nursing homes, the type of cushion on which the individual sits during the day should be written in the care plan.

Cushions

Cushions can be made of a variety of materials including silicore, foam, gel, fluid and air (Figs 11.9 and 11.10). Depending on the material used and their construction, cushions will be suitable for different levels of risk. In nursing homes the registered nurse will ensure that the cushions provided are suitable for the individual patients. In residential homes, you can obtain advice from district nursing staff.

Silicore cushions are padded cushions covered in fabric. They are used for comfort only. They can be machine washed and dried. Some have a waterproof side or seat that can be wiped clean. Special silicore cushions are designed to fit into wheelchairs. Armchairs with integral pressure reducing cushions are now available (Fig. 11.11).

Foam cushions come in varying densities and can be made of different kinds of foam. They are light and simple to use. Some have a moulded surface that helps the cushion conform better to

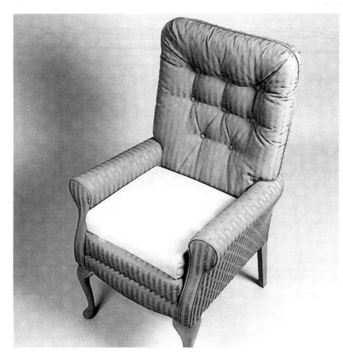

Fig. 11.9 Pressure reducing foam cushion.

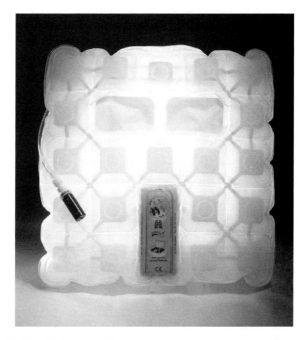

Fig. 11.10 Airtech cushion.

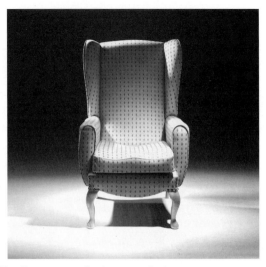

Fig. 11.11   Pressure reducing armchair.

body shape and reduces shear. Some have a special core that allows air to circulate and prevents heat building up.

Gel cushions may be solid or fluid and are sometimes combined with foam to make them lighter. Fluid cushions can also be filled with foam in a way that has a dampening effect on the flow of fluid or to provide support for a fluid filled pad.

Alternating air cushions (Fig. 11.12) are designed to relieve pressure from the seating surface. Like pressure relieving mattresses their cells inflate and deflate in sequence to either support or relieve pressure from this area. They are either mains operated or powered by battery packs.

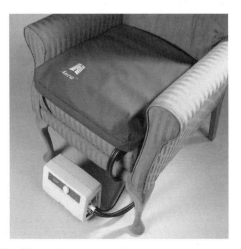

Fig. 11.12   Alternating air cushion.

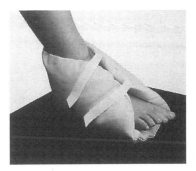

Fig. 11.13   Heel protectors.

Heel protectors

Heel protectors (Fig. 11.13) are aids used to protect the heels of people who are very frail and at high risk of developing pressure sores. They are made of either sheepskin (real or synthetic) or silicore fibre, and are held in place with Velcro straps. They help reduce and relieve pressure.

Heel blocks are made of soft foam and have a U shape in the middle. The ankle fits into the U shape and the heels are held up and do not touch the mattress. Heel blocks can only be used when the person is sitting up or lying on his back. Heel protectors are used when the person is lying on his side.

Elbow protectors

Elbow protectors (Fig. 11.14) are designed to protect elbows. They are also made of sheepskin or silicore and are held in place with Velcro straps.

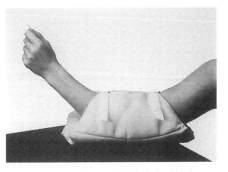

Fig. 11.14   Elbow protectors.

Treating pressure sores

If you fear that a person is developing a pressure sore, you should always seek professional help and advice. In most cases, nurses will be responsible for treating the pressure sore. The nurse will assess the sore and plan treatment and care. This will include changing the person's position regularly; special mattresses, cushions and pressure-relieving aids may be used. The pressure sore will be covered with a protective dressing to keep the wound clean and prevent it from drying out. Wounds of all types, including pressure sores, are now known to heal more quickly if they are kept warm and moist. You will be involved in helping carry out the plan of care.

Caring for the whole person

People develop pressure sores because they are unable to move and relieve pressure. Illness can make a person more at risk of developing a pressure sore and the patient's doctor will treat any illness that could contribute to the development of a pressure sore.

If pressure sores are to be prevented it is important that the individual eats a healthy diet and has sufficient food and vitamins to prevent the skin breaking down. Older people who feel unwell may be reluctant to eat. It is important that you inform senior staff if an individual has gone off their food. You can also find out what food the older person is fond of and inform other members of staff about their likes and dislikes.

It is important that the individual drinks enough fluid. You can encourage the older person to drink and can ensure that they have drinks that they like. You can inform other members of staff about the individual's likes and dislikes. Further details on diet and fluids are given in Chapter 6.

Summary

Older people are more at risk of developing pressure sores than younger people. People living in homes are more at risk than those who live in their own homes. Pressure sores are at best uncomfortable and painful; at their worst they can be life threatening. Most pressure sores can be prevented.

Some people living in homes are more frail than others. Assessment enables nurses to work out the individual's degree of risk of developing pressure sores, and to develop a plan of care.

This enables the nurse to decide which type of mattresses, cushions and aids are required. The nurse should discuss the plan of care with the individual and obtain their consent and co-operation. You are an important part of the team. You need to be aware of the plan of care and should work with senior staff to prevent individuals developing pressure sores.

Portfolio preparation

Your assessor must have evidence that you can meet the performance criteria for this unit. Before beginning this unit discuss assessment strategies with your assessor. Most of the evidence for this unit can be gained by direct observation of your work. You may be asked to provide the following types of evidence:

■ Products. This might include a copy of progress notes or a care plan on pressure area care that you have completed. Remember to delete the resident's name to preserve confidentiality.
■ Witness testimony. This is a statement from a senior member of staff. It might be a statement detailing how you have met certain performance criteria.
■ Written work. You might be asked to prepare a piece of work about the factors that increase the risk of pressure sores developing.

Your assessor may also use other methods to help you gain evidence for this unit. These may include:

■ Verbal questioning
■ Written questions
■ Watching you prepare pressure relieving equipment such as an alternating pressure overlay. Watching you demonstrate how a particular piece of pressure relieving equipment is used.

Further information

You can obtain leaflets and further information on wound care and preventing pressure sores from the companies listed below.

Convatec
Harrington House
Milton Road
Ickenham
Uxbridge UB10 8PU
Help-line Tel. 0800 289738
Convatec produce a useful booklet, *Pressure Sore Blueprint*. This is available free of charge. They also run a wound care help-line.

Coloplast
Peterborough Business Park
Peterborough
Cambs PE2 6FX
Tel. 01733 392000

Johnson & Johnson Medical
Coronation Road
Ascot
Berkshire SL5 9EY
Tel. 01344 871000

Pharma-plast Limited
Steriseal Division
Thornhill Road
Redditch
Worcester B98 9NL
Tel. 01527 64222

Smith & Nephew Healthcare
S&N Healthcare House
Goulton Street
Hull HU3 4DJ
Tel. 01482 222200

Huntleigh Healthcare
310–312 Dallow Road
Luton
Bedfordshire LU1 1TD
Tel. 01582 413104

Chapter 12

Personal Care and Hygiene

Introduction

This chapter provides information on the option group A units Z9, Z9.1 and Z9.2 – 'enable clients to maintain their personal hygiene and appearance'.

This chapter provides information on:

- Bathing
- Making bathing a pleasure
- Persuading the reluctant resident to bath
- Using hoists
- Safety and privacy in the bathroom
- Showers, assisted washes and bedbaths
- Skin care, including skin care for incontinent residents and the use of barrier creams
- Mouth care including care of dentures and natural teeth
- Nail care including chiropody treatment
- Hair care and hairdressing
- Shaving
- Choosing clothing and dressing
- Cosmetics

Looking good and feeling good

People of all ages like to feel and look good. Many older people who have been in hospital arrive in homes wearing night-clothes and looking ill and tired. When the person is dressed in her normal clothes, has her hair set and is wearing make-up, she feels and looks much better. When we feel dirty, untidy and under the weather, bathing and making the effort to look good make us feel so much better.

Many older people who have just undergone surgery, for example for a fractured femur, feel worn out and fed up. Often they are unable to wash, dress and care for themselves without help. The care assistant can make a real difference to the person's quality of life. You can encourage and assist the older person to bath, to care for her hair and nails and to dress. This can make a real difference to the individual's morale. Suddenly the experience of coming into a home is not as bad as the individual feared. She is being helped to care for herself and is beginning to feel human again. It has been said that the role of the nurse is to do for the patient what they would do for themselves if they had the strength and the will. Helping people to care for their personal appearance is not about helping residents to look or appear as we would wish, but as they would wish.

Bathing

Nowadays most of us take bathrooms and their supply of constant hot water for granted. Many older people, though, grew up without such luxuries. They grew up in homes without bathrooms, central heating or hot water. People who did not have bathrooms either heated up water and bathed in a tin bath in front of a fire in the living room, or they visited the public baths. This involved much more effort than going upstairs and running a bath and so many older people bathed much less frequently than we do now.

How often a person baths is a personal choice. Some older people prefer to bath each day, while others feel that bathing twice a week is adequate. Bathing every day can help some residents to feel fresh and clean, for example those who perspire heavily or who suffer from incontinence. No harm, however, will come to most people if they do not bath every day. The decision on how often to bath should be the older person's. While you can persuade an older person to bath, no older person should be bullied into bathing if they do not wish to do so. Bathing should be a pleasure and not a hurried chore. If you take the time and trouble to make the person's bath a pleasant experience you will find that the older person will look forward to the next bath.

Making bathing a pleasure

Many older people living in homes require help to bath. Even people who can bath without help depend on us to ensure that the bathroom is safe, warm and comfortable. In some homes bathrooms become used as storerooms and fill up with boxes, broken chairs, commodes and other equipment. You should do everything you can to make sure that the bathroom is not used as a storeroom. Imagine how you would feel bathing in a room full of junk. Ask senior staff if equipment can be stored elsewhere.

Keeping the bathroom clear makes it less likely that residents and staff will have an accident in the bathroom.

Often the bathroom window is left open and the room becomes cold. You should check that the window is closed before running the bath. The bathroom radiator should be turned on. If you find the bathroom hot, remember that the person who has just got out of the bath will find it much cooler.

The bath water should be the correct temperature. You should ask the individual how they like the water. Many hot water taps in homes are thermostatically controlled to prevent scalding but valves can become defective. It is better to be safe than sorry. Check the water temperature with an elbow before helping a resident into the bath. In some homes bath thermometers are still used but these are becoming less common as homes switch to thermostatically controlled valves. People who are confused may be unable to tell you if the water is too hot. Residents who have no feeling in part of their body may not feel water that is too hot. In 1998, 30 older people in hospital, nursing and residential homes suffered from serious burns because the water they were bathing in was too hot.

The water should be deep enough to wash in. Some staff attempt to bath residents in a few inches of water.

Bubble baths and bath oils

Many people like to use scented bubble bath or bath oils in the bath. Bubble bath adds a touch of luxury and many people enjoy using it. Some bubble baths, though, can make an older person's skin very dry; moisturising cream bubble bath can prevent this. Some older people have very sensitive skin and bubble bath can make it itch. It is now possible to buy bubble baths especially for people with sensitive skin. These avoid using agents such as lanolin, which can cause allergies. Most supermarkets sell their own brand of sensitive skin bubble bath and many other companies make them too. You can either ask relatives to buy these, can buy them for the older person who can pay from their personal allowance, or can take the older person shopping. This will depend on the policy of the home. Some older people continue to suffer from dry or sensitive skin despite these measures and you should seek professional advice. The person's doctor may prescribe special bubble bath designed for people with very sensitive skin.

Bath oils should be used with caution. Some make the skin very slippery. This does not normally cause a problem if the older person is helped in and out of the bath by using a hoist. If the individual only requires a hand to step out of the bath then bath oils that can make the skin, the bath and even a bath mat slippery, should be used with care.

Soap

Some older people prefer to wash with soap instead of using bubble bath, shower gel and foam washes. Most people can use soap without any ill effects. Some older people who have dry skin find that soap makes it even drier. It is now possible to buy soaps that have moisturising cream in them; using these prevents the skin becoming dry. People with sensitive skin can use unperfumed soaps made specially for sensitive skins. If these do not help, the person's doctor can prescribe special soap. Some older people especially those with eczema may, on doctor's advice, wash using emulsifying ointment instead of soap.

Talcum powder

Many older people like to use talcum powder after drying their skin. Some older people may find that heavily perfumed talc makes their skin itch. Using either baby powder or unscented talcum powder can prevent this problem.

Persuading the reluctant resident to bath

Some older people may be reluctant to bath. They may have found that the bath was rushed and was an ordeal rather than a pleasure. Male residents may be embarrassed to appear naked in front of a young female care assistant. Some older people need help to get in and out of the bath but may not like to ask as they do not want to 'appear a nuisance' or 'trouble the staff'. Some older people may be suffering from pain and may fear that getting in and out of the bath will make it worse. Others may feel that there is no opportunity to bath in private. You should take the time and trouble to find out why the older person is reluctant and should try to make bathing as pleasant an experience as possible.

If the person likes a long leisurely soak but the bathrooms are busy in the morning, perhaps you could suggest a bath in the afternoon or evening when the home is not so busy. If the individual does not wish to bath, you should respect the person's wishes.

Case history

Mrs Eltringham was admitted to the Hollies from hospital. She had refused to bath in hospital and was described as 'difficult'. Mrs Eltringham's key worker Joanne Davies spent time with Mrs

Eltringham. She discovered that Mrs Eltringham was terrified of bathing. A year before she had slipped in the bath at home. She broke her arm, was unable to get out and spent several hours alone and afraid in the bath before her daughter visited and found her. Joanne suggested that Mrs Eltringham try a shower and Mrs Eltringham agreed.

Using hoists – legal requirements

Hoists are often used to help frail older people get in and out of the bath safely. Many people living in homes need help to get in and out of the bath. Some people merely require a steadying hand; others are unable to stand, bend or get into the bath unless they are lifted.

In the past, staff in some homes were expected to lift older people in and out of the bath without hoists. Sometimes, if an individual was very disabled or heavy, two people had to lift the individual out. Many bathrooms are small. Staff often had difficulty in lifting because there was not enough room. Staff were in danger of injuring their backs and at risk of injuring the resident.

In January 1993, six European Community directives were introduced to improve health and safety. The Manual Handling Loads Directive states that:

'The employer shall have a duty to ensure the safety and health of all workers in every aspect of work'.

Under UK and European law, employers have a duty to introduce policies to assess the risk of injury if staff lift people or objects. Homes should have policies that assess all manual handling operations and identify the risk of injury.

A hoist should be used to bath people who are unable to bear any of their own weight. Employers who expect staff to lift residents in and out of the bath and do not provide hoists are acting illegally.

Two different types of hoist are normally used to enable people to bath. The first is a mobile hoist, which is normally on wheels and is wheeled to the person (Fig. 12.1). The person is transferred onto the hoist and wheeled to the bathroom. The hoist is attached to an upright column that is screwed to the floor and the hoist is raised off the ground by turning a handle. The section of the hoist that has the wheels is detached, and the chair section is placed over the bath. The person is lowered into the bath.

The second type is a fixed hoist. This is a chair with a lifting column and a base plate screwed to the floor (Fig. 12.2). The person walks or is wheeled into the bathroom, and is then helped

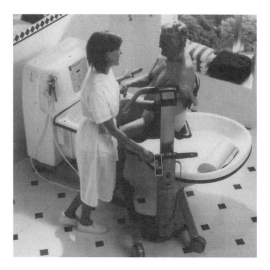

Fig. 12.1   Mobile hoist.

to transfer into the hoist. The hoist is raised and positioned over the bath, and the person is lowered into the bath.

Fixed hoists are suitable for residents who are more able. The disadvantage of fixed hoists is that an individual who requires help to transfer must be transferred from chair to wheelchair to hoist and then back again. Using a mobile hoist reduces the number of transfers required. Mobile hoists, though, can cost three times as much as fixed hoists. They also take up more room. In homes that

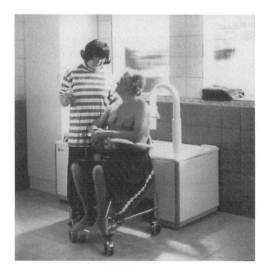

Fig. 12.2   Fixed hoist.

have not been purpose built, bathrooms are often small and there may not be enough room for a mobile hoist. Well designed bathing facilities can enable people with disabilities to bath unaided (Fig. 12.3).

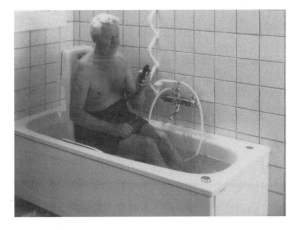

Fig. 12.3 Bathing aids can be used to enable people to bath unaided.

Few residential homes have mobile hoists because people are less disabled than those in nursing homes. Nursing homes should have facilities for bathing very disabled residents. A mobile hoist or a special type of bath such as a Parker bath (Fig. 12.4) should be provided. Using special equipment such as hoists and Parker baths protects both residents and staff from injury. You should check

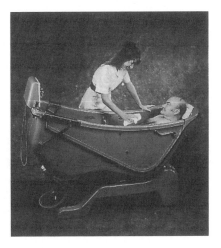

Fig. 12.4 Parker bath.

which types of hoists are available in your workplace and make sure you know how to operate them. Details of equipment required to lift the individual who cannot bear part of his or her weight should be written on the care plan.

Further information on moving and handling is given in Chapter 10.

Safety and privacy in the bathroom

Most people expect to enjoy a bath in peace without interruptions. Most people lock the bathroom door and enjoy a relaxing bath. How many residents in homes can enjoy peace and privacy while bathing? In some homes staff leave the bathroom door ajar so that they can 'keep an eye on' the older person. In other homes staff have strict instructions that residents must not be left alone in the bathroom, 'in the interests of safety'. Yet the nursing or residential home is the person's home and all over the country older people bath without being watched.

Some people, though, are very frail and it would not be safe to leave them alone. Some individuals who suffer from dementia and are confused could try to get up and could fall, or could slip over and drown. In 1999, 20 people were injured while bathing in hospitals and homes.

How can staff respect the person's privacy and dignity and yet prevent accidents? It is important to realise that very few older people are at risk of injuring themselves while bathing. Staff have a duty of care and any member of staff who left a resident unattended in the bath knowing that the resident was at risk of injury would have failed in that duty of care. Older people living in homes have differing abilities. An older person who lives in a home and who requires assistance to get in and out of the bath has the same right to privacy as a person living in their own home. If the older person can be safely left in the bath then everyone should respect the individual's right to privacy.

However, if the older person is confused and in danger of injuring herself, you would be failing to provide proper care if you failed to remain with the person. If the person suffers from a disease that may cause her to faint or lose consciousness, you should remain with the person to ensure that she is safe.

In nursing homes, the care plan should include details of how much assistance the individual requires and what measures are required to maintain safety. If you are not sure check with senior staff. The charity Counsel and Care have produced a book about balancing resident safety and providing dignity and privacy (Counsel & Care 1993).

Showers

Many new homes have specially designed shower rooms. Unfortunately, many of these shower rooms are seldom used. Many older people are reluctant to use showers because they have not used them before. Many staff who have worked in older homes without showers prefer not to use showers.

Showers can be refreshing. Modern specially designed showers enable older people to wash themselves. Some showers are in specially designed rooms with slightly sloping floors. Special shower seats are provided so that the individual can shower sitting down. Often shower controls have been placed at sitting height and the showers have thermostatic valves to prevent scalding. Shower chairs with wheels are available so that the person who cannot walk can be wheeled into the shower room where she can shower or be helped to shower.

Some showers are not purpose built and resemble ordinary shower cubicles. Placing a plastic chair in the cubicle, such as the type of stacking chair homes often provide for visits, can enable people who are unable to stand to use the shower. Showers should have non-slip flooring, but even some of this can become quite slippery when wet. You should help older people who are in danger of slipping, when they are going in and out of the shower. If the shower does not have a thermostatic valve that prevents the risk of scalding, you should adjust the water temperature and remain with the person to check that the water does not get too hot.

Soap can be difficult to keep hold of in the shower, especially for older people who may have suffered from strokes or have arthritic hands. Soap on a rope can be hooked around the shower control (if at sitting height) or on a hook, to make washing easier. Some residents prefer to use shower gels or body washes that can also be used as shampoos. These are available in sensitive skin and non-perfumed versions for people who have dry and sensitive skin. People who have difficulty gripping a flannel can find it difficult to wash independently using soap and a flannel. One solution is to squeeze shower gel onto a nylon beauty buff (such as that made by Oil of Olay) as this can be used one handed.

Assisted washes

Individuals who do not wish to bath or shower each day may need help to wash. They may need help to get soap, flannels, talc, deodorant and clothing ready. If everything is ready before the wash, the water will not get cold. You can help the person to the wash basin and help them to wash. It is safer for most older people to wash sitting in a chair.

The wash basin may be too high to allow the person to use it comfortably when seated. In this case, you can bring a bowl of warm water. The person remains seated in the chair and the water is placed on a bed table. It is important to make sure that the person is able to wash in private. If the person shares a room with another person, curtains should be drawn. If the room is over-looked, the window curtains should be drawn. If the person has a single room it may have a 'Do not disturb' or 'Engaged' sign on the outside; this should be used so that visitors do not enter and embarrass the person who is washing.

The individual may require help to undress. You should encourage the person to wash as much of the body as they can manage. Often older people who require assisted washes find it difficult to wash the back, bottom, lower legs and feet. You can wash these areas, dry them thoroughly, and apply powder if the person uses it. Then help put on any clothing that the individual is unable to manage.

Bed baths

People who are very frail and ill may require a bed bath. This is simply a name for a wash that is carried out in bed. It may be carried out by one or two members of staff depending on the home's policies, staffing levels and how much care the resident requires.

Towels, flannels, soap, talcum powder, deodorant and any other toiletries are removed from the person's locker, with the person's permission, and placed on the bed table. A bowl of water is brought to the bedside. The bed curtains are drawn, the room door closed and window curtains drawn if the room is overlooked. You must explain that you intend to wash the person and make her more comfortable.

The bedclothes or duvet are removed and the person is covered with a sheet, blanket or large towel depending on the home's policy and the temperature. If it is a hot sticky summer's day, a blanket could be hot and uncomfortable. On a chilly winter's morning, a sheet would not be warm enough. Two flannels are used for washing. One, usually a light colour, is used for the face. Another, usually a darker colour, is used for the body. Many people, especially women, do not use soap on their faces and only wash the face with plain water. You should ask the person if she normally washes her face with soap.

You then fold the cover back and wash the neck, arms, chest

and abdomen. The flannel is soaped and an area of the body washed. The flannel is then rinsed and the area of the body rinsed and dried. Apply deodorant or antiperspirant if the person wishes. Apply talcum powder if the person wishes. It is easy to use too much talcum powder if using it directly from the container. This can be uncomfortable and can cause skin irritation. If too much talcum powder is used in skin folds, such as under the arms or under the breasts, the powder can cake. Placing talcum powder on a powder puff and then applying it to the skin prevents this, as it is easier to avoid putting too much on. Supermarkets and chemists sell powder puffs designed for applying talc.

If the person can sit forward, ask her to do so and wash her back. People who are able to do so should be encouraged to wash their own genital area. If the person is unable to assist by sitting up, a second member of staff can help lie the person down and roll her over onto her side. Staff should explain what they are going to do and obtain consent before moving her. The front of the body is covered and the back, buttocks and the area between the legs (perineum) is washed and dried. The person may like to have powder on her back.

It is not advisable to put powder on the perineal area or the groin as the powder can cake. This is a particular problem with people who are incontinent and people who sweat a lot. If the person is incontinent, a barrier cream may be applied lightly to the buttocks and perineum. Too much cream interferes with the action of incontinence pads. Further details on caring for the skin of incontinent residents is given later in this chapter.

The water should then be changed. This is important because the water will have become cooler and full of soap suds. The back of the legs are then washed and the person is rolled over onto her back. The top half of the person's body is covered and the remaining parts of the lower front of the body washed and dried and powder applied if the person wishes.

Some staff prefer to turn the person onto her back before changing the water. This practice will vary depending on the person's condition. A person with breathing difficulties will find it easier to breathe if sat up, whilst other people may be safer left on their sides. Some staff prefer to lift and wash the front of the leg and then lift it to wash the back. This again will depend on the person's condition, as this can be uncomfortable for people who have arthritis. Although techniques vary, the basic principles remain the same. It is important to protect the person's dignity at all times. You must ensure that the person's body remains covered and that only the part being washed is exposed.

The person is then dressed or helped to dress in clean clothes. If the person is well enough she can be helped to sit in a chair while bed linen is changed and the bed made. You can then help the person to clean teeth or dentures, to comb and style hair, and to apply make-up if she wishes. Male residents may require help with shaving.

In some homes, you may find that the bed bathing technique varies. Some staff use two bowls of water to carry out a bed bath, one for washing and the other for rinsing. Both bowls of water will still require changing, as the water will become cooler.

It is important to remember that although bed bathing techniques differ, the aims remain the same. The person's dignity and privacy should be protected at all times. The person should be covered to prevent her from becoming cold. The person's own preferences should be sought. One important part of bed bathing is sometimes forgotten – the person being bed bathed. Bed bathing a person gives you the opportunity to get to know the person and to communicate with her. Often people confide their worries and fears during a bed bath. A resident may tell you that her arthritis seems to be getting worse and that the pain killers do not seem to be doing so much good these days.

Another might confide that the new tablets make her feel sick. It is important that you share such information with senior staff. The doctor may be able to change the pain killers or increase the dose so that the person is no longer in pain. The person whose tablets are making her feel sick may be able to have a different type of tablets.

Skin care

Skin is a waterproof protective covering. It is sensitive to heat, cold, touch and pressure. Skin is elastic and stretches, and it grows and contracts as a person becomes fatter or thinner. Healthy skin protects the body against infection. As people age, their skin becomes less elastic and tends to wrinkle. The skin becomes drier and thinner and can be more easily damaged than the skin of younger people. Certain medicines, such as steroids and anti-inflammatory drugs given to treat arthritis, affect the skin. These medicines can cause the skin to be very easily damaged.

When the skin is damaged, it is no longer able to prevent infection. Dry skin can become damaged more easily than healthy skin. Many older people suffer from very dry skin, and it is usually worst on the legs and arms. Older people's skin is often more sensitive than younger people's. You should advise older people with sensitive and dry skin to avoid using heavily perfumed soaps and bubble baths. Special moisturising bubble baths and soaps can now be bought in most supermarkets and chemists.

Caring for dry skin

People who have dry skin may have found their own solutions. Some people have their own favourite moisturisers that they have been using for years. Sometimes the older person is no longer able to bend down and apply moisturiser to the legs or another part of the body. You should offer to do this if the older person can no longer manage.

Sometimes the skin is so dry that normal moisturisers and oils are not effective. In this case, seek professional advice. The person's doctor may prescribe special moisturising creams. These should normally be applied after a bath. Some creams are more effective if applied to damp skin. Registered nurses will be able to offer advice and show you how to apply these moisturising creams. People who require specially prescribed creams should have this noted in their care plan in nursing homes. A record should also be kept in residential homes. Care assistants who are applying these creams will soon see if the prescribed cream is effective. You should inform professional staff and colleagues about the condition of the person's skin. If the skin is not improving the doctor will visit again and may prescribe a different cream. In very severe cases, the person's doctor may ask a skin specialist or dermatologist to see the person.

Caring for the skin of incontinent people

People who suffer from incontinence can easily develop inflamed skin (dermatitis) because the skin is in contact with urine. People who are incontinent of faeces as well as urine are at high risk of developing sore inflamed skin. This inflamed skin can become infected and can increase the risk of developing pressure sores. People who are incontinent should be washed each time they have been incontinent. Washing removes traces of urine from the skin. Urine can irritate the skin and cause soreness.

Many people who are incontinent have their genital area and bottom washed six or seven times each day. If you use soap each time, the skin can soon become very dry. Dry skin can develop small cracks and can easily become infected. You can avoid this by using soap and water only two or three times each day. The soap used should be mild and unperfumed. At other times use plain water to clean the skin. If the person prefers to use soap then use a soap with moisturiser.

Barrier creams – are they necessary?

Barrier creams are creams that are used to coat the skin and provide a protective barrier that prevents the skin becoming soggy and sore. Some nurses who specialise in the care of people with continence problems (continence advisers) state that barrier creams should only be used if the person's skin is becoming sore. Others state that prevention is better than cure. Many registered nurses disagree on when barrier creams should be used.

Anyone who is incontinent of faeces and urine should have a barrier cream applied at all times. This will help prevent the skin becoming sore when faeces and urine mix to form ammonia, which can cause skin damage very quickly. Anyone who has red, inflamed skin should have a barrier cream applied. In the home where I work barrier cream is routinely applied to the bottom and genital area of all residents who suffer from incontinence. Skin problems are rare.

Which barrier cream is best?

There are more than 50 different barrier creams available. Some continence advisers recommend using petroleum jelly. This forms a waterproof barrier and stops urine sticking to the skin. Others recommend zinc and castor oil cream and others will recommend different preparations. People are individuals and a cream that is effective and protects one person's skin may not be so effective on another person's skin. Many homes use a few different products. These are prescribed by the doctor for the individual. Each person who requires a barrier cream should have his or her own labelled cream, which should be used only for that person. Sharing or borrowing creams increases the risk of infection. If an individual's skin is becoming sore or is failing to improve despite a cream being used, you should seek professional advice. The individual may have developed a skin infection (cellulitis), and prompt treatment can prevent further complications from developing.

Mouth care

Mouth care is an area of caring that is often forgotten, carried out poorly or thought to be of little importance. Mouth care, though, is very important. The person who has a toothache, sore gums because dentures are rubbing or a sore tongue because a broken tooth is catching on it, may not wish to eat or drink. Without sufficient food and fluids, the person will become weaker and less able to fight off illness. A sore mouth can make a person feel miserable and depressed. It has been said that the best way of judging the quality of care is to check the mouths of residents.

Caring for natural teeth

Many older people living in homes no longer have any natural teeth. Some older people, though, have some or all of their own teeth. People admitted to nursing homes will have a nursing history taken before they are admitted. This will have information about the person's teeth, dentures or partial dentures written on it. In residential homes, you may have to enquire.

People who have their own teeth should care for them normally. The teeth should be brushed morning and evening; some forgetful residents may need reminding. People who are unable to walk to the wash basin will require a tooth mug with water, a dish to rinse their mouths into, and their toothbrush and toothpaste. Some older people are unable to brush their teeth and you may have to do it for them. Try practising by brushing a colleague's teeth. You can then swap roles and discuss it when you have finished.

People who have their natural teeth should continue to have six-monthly dental check-ups and may require dental treatment such as fillings and crowns. Dental check-ups can be carried out either at the dental surgery or at the home. Dentists who provide dental care to the home may be either dentists who practice locally or part of the community dental service. Find out what the dental arrangements are in your home.

As people age, their teeth are more at risk of breaking or cracking. People who have their own teeth should be advised not to eat hard sweets such as boiled sweets and sugared almonds, as crunching on these can cause teeth to break. Toffees and eclairs can sometimes cause loose fillings to come out.

Caring for dentures

Caring for dentures is as important as caring for natural teeth. People who are unable to clean their dentures can have food debris building up under them. This can cause gums to become sore and inflamed. Dentures should be cleaned morning and evening with a toothbrush and toothpaste. Some older people do not remove dentures but clean them while they are in the mouth. It is not possible to clean the inner part of the dentures or the top palate without removing them. Individuals should be advised to remove dentures so that they can be cleaned properly.

Many older people prefer to remove dentures and soak them overnight. Dentures can be soaked in either plain water or denture cleaning tablets. Recent research reveals that dentures can become heavily contaminated with bacteria. These bacteria can cause sore mouths, gums and throats. Using denture cleaning tablets after thorough cleaning destroys these harmful bacteria. The denture pot is filled with warm water and the denture-cleaning tablet is added. Cleaned dentures are soaked overnight. Denture cleaning tablets contain a mild bleach and this removes stains such as coffee and tea. It can be difficult to remove such stains by brushing. Badly stained dentures or dentures with a visible build up of tartar can be professionally cleaned by the dentist. If an older person who wears dentures complains of sore gums, professional advice should be sought. The denture may have become ill fitting and is rubbing. The dentist can treat this and adjust, alter, or make new dentures if required.

Mouth care for the frail older person

People who are very ill or frail may depend on staff to clean their mouths. Many older people who are unwell are unable to tolerate their dentures. The person who feels sick may find having the dentures out is more comfortable. Other people prefer to continue to wear their dentures. Denture care is as given above.

The frail person should be offered mouthwashes. There are many different types available. Dentists now recommend that plain water is offered as a mouthwash. Mouthwashes, research has discovered, can kill off bacteria in the mouth that keep the mouth healthy. Using mouthwashes can cause sore mouths and some individuals can develop oral thrush if they are used. Normally, unless a mouthwash has been especially prescribed by the person's doctor or dentist, the mouth is only rinsed with plain water.

Some people are so ill and frail that they are unable to rinse their mouths with water. Some homes have mouth care trays, which have special swabs to clean out the mouth. These are sticks with a piece of pink foam on top. The foam is dipped into water and then inserted into the person's mouth. Some homes no longer use these. There have been cases where the foam has come off the stick or has been bitten off. The foam has been inhaled in a few cases and emergency hospital treatment required to remove the foam from the lung. In some homes pre-moistened swabs that resemble giant cotton buds are available. There have been no reports of problems with their use.

The aim of mouth care is to remove food debris and traces of milky fluids from the mouth. Dentists now recommend that gauze moistened in water is wrapped around a gloved finger and used to gently clean the mouth. The inside of the mouth can be wiped with glycerine after cleaning. This keeps the mouth moist and prevents soreness. Lips can become dry, sore and cracked when people are very ill. Petroleum jelly or lip salve prevents this and keeps the individual feeling comfortable.

Nail care

Many older people have difficulty in caring for their nails. People who suffer from arthritis can find it difficult to use scissors or nail clippers because their hands can no longer manage fine movements. People with poor eyesight cannot see well enough to cut or file nails. People suffering from Parkinson's disease often suffer from fine tremors that make nail care difficult. People who have suffered from strokes and can only use one hand find it impossible to care for their nails. One survey of fit and healthy people over the age of 85 found that few people of this age could manage to bend down and cut their own toenails.

Uncared for fingernails can become dirty and torn and people with nails like this look uncared for and dishevelled. Many people prefer to have their nails cut with nail scissors or clippers and kept short. Some women though prefer to keep their nails longer and have them filed, manicured and painted with nail varnish. You should ask individuals how they prefer to have their fingernails and should not assume that all older women like short nails.

Case history

Grace Adams felt depressed when she had to give up her home and enter a nursing home. Her key worker noticed that her nails were long and dirty and offered to attend to them. Grace explained that she had always been proud of her hands and nails and had kept her nails long, manicured and painted red all of her adult life. Having attractive hands and nails made her feel feminine and attractive. One of the things that had upset her most was that she was unable to care for her hands and paint her nails after her stroke. Her carer, June, soaked her hands in a bowl of water, scrubbed the dirt from beneath her nails, and pushed back the ragged cuticles surrounding the nails with a Cutipen. She applied hand cream to the hands, painted Grace's nails with two coats of nail varnish, and applied a top coat of varnish. Grace felt like an attractive woman again and not a 'dishevelled old dear with dirty nails'. Caring for the person's nails can have an important effect on morale. You get a great feeling of satisfaction from making a person feel better.

Many older people are unable to cut their own toenails and many are admitted to homes with nails that have become so long they are curling over and cutting into the toes. Some older people have toenails that are very thick and difficult to cut. Toenails become thicker when circulation to the feet is poor. It is almost impossible to cut thickened toenails with ordinary nail scissors. Older people who do not have thickened toenails can have their toenails cut with ordinary nail scissors. You should check what the policy is for cutting the nails of people who have thickened toenails. In some nursing homes, these nails are cut by registered nurses. The home should have strong nail scissors, clippers and files so that these nails can be cut. In other homes, RNs do not cut nails but arrange for the chiropodist to call and do it.

Chiropodists

Many chiropodists work with foot care assistants and will often arrange for a foot care assistant to come to the home and cut nails. Chiropodists will call and treat residents who have foot problems such as ingrowing toenails, corns and bunions. The chiropodist who visits the home may be either a private chiropodist or one employed by the local NHS community trust. Private chiropodists charge either by the session (usually three quarters of an hour) or charge for each resident seen. If your home uses a private chiropodist find out how much each treatment costs. In most homes individuals pay these charges as they are seldom included in home fees except in the most expensive of private homes. There is no charge for NHS chiropody but some areas do not have enough chiropody staff and it can be difficult to arrange regular visits.

Hair care

As people age, the hair loses the pigment that gives us our hair colour. Hair becomes grey or white. White hair is coarser in texture and drier. Hair thins with age. Men may lose all their hair and become bald. The scalp becomes drier and more sensitive with age. Older people very rarely have greasy hair and usually a shampoo once or twice each week will keep the hair clean. Washing the hair daily will make dry hair and a dry scalp even drier. Older people should be encouraged or helped to wash their hair once or twice a week. If the hair is dry, a mild shampoo for dry hair should be used. Many older women have their hair permed regularly. Perming makes the hair dry. Residents who have perms should use a conditioner after shampooing, to prevent the hair becoming dry and brittle and make it easier to comb and style. Some people prefer to use a shampoo and conditioner in one. If this is used then one specially for dry hair should be chosen.

If a person is unwell and unable to have a shampoo, a dry shampoo can be used to freshen up the hair. Dry shampoos can be purchased in chemists and are powders that are puffed onto the hair through an applicator and then brushed out. They remove dirt and debris from the hair but do not tire a person out when she is feeling unwell. Dry shampoos are not intended to be used long term. They can be useful if someone is feeling under the weather, perhaps because of a chest infection or an illness.

Some older people develop dry, flaking and itching scalps; in extreme cases, sores can form on the scalp and these can bleed. If an individual develops a dry, flaking, itchy scalp, professional advice should be sought. The person's doctor will normally pre-scribe a shampoo containing coal tar (to prevent the flaking and treat the itching) and coconut oil (to treat the dryness). The hair is normally shampooed daily and the shampoo left on for 10–15 minutes; as the condition improves the hair is washed less fre-quently, until it is washed once or twice each week. These shampoos can dry the hair terribly and a rich conditioner should be applied after use. Perming lotions, tints and setting lotions should not be used until the doctor has agreed that the scalp is normal. The hairdresser should be informed about any problems with a person's scalp and will test each lotion on the individual's forearm to make sure that the person is not allergic to it, before using it on the person's hair.

Hairdressing

For many women a trip to the hairdressers is a treat. Women feel good when their hair looks good. Having a hairdo is important to many older women. Most homes have a hairdresser who visits once or twice a week and washes, cuts, perms, shampoos and sets hair for female residents. Male residents have their hair cut.

It is important to realise that women do not stop caring about their appearance as they age. You can help residents keep their hair looking nice between styles. Some people have fine hair and find that wearing a hairnet helps keep a set looking good for longer. You can help the individual put on her hairnet before going to sleep if she can no longer manage this. When you are helping the individual to wash and dress remember to help comb and style hair if the person has difficulty.

Shaving

Men, especially older men, often feel dirty and scruffy if they are unshaven. Many male residents have difficulty shaving. A stroke can cause an older person to lose the use of one hand. Parkinson's disease can cause tremor. Poor eyesight can make it difficult to see well enough to shave.

Wet shaves

Many older men prefer to use a shaving stick and brush to make shaving foam. This is applied to the bristles to soften the hair. Shaving foam may contain perfume and people with sensitive skin can react to this and suffer from red and itchy skin. It is now possible to buy shaving sticks, foam and gel for sensitive skin. A razor is then used to remove hair.

Using a foam and a razor gives a closer shave then using an electric razor, and many older men prefer a wet shave. Many care assistants fear cutting the person's skin and encourage the individual (or his relatives) to buy an electric razor. Wet shaving is not difficult (half of the adult population do it daily). It is a skill that is easily learnt. If a male resident prefers to have a wet shave, respect the individual's wishes. Senior staff can help and advise you in learning how to shave a male resident.

Electric razors

Many male residents, including those who have a tremor or can only use one hand, find it possible to shave using an electric razor. Electric razors can help an older person retain his independence. Each male resident should have his own razor. You should not 'borrow' another resident's electric razor for someone whose own shaver is broken. Electric razors can cause very small cuts on the skin. If two people share a razor, there is a risk of both developing a skin infection.

After-shave

Many men like to use after-shave, but it contains perfume, alcohol and colourings and these can inflame the skin of some people. Special after-shave made for people with sensitive skin can be used if ordinary after-shave irritates the skin.

Clothing

Our clothes say a lot about us, about our personality and our mood. Older people enjoy wearing clothes that they have chosen themselves. Clothing should be comfortable, attractive and practical. Many older people living in homes enjoy choosing their own clothes, yet in many homes clothes are not chosen and bought by the individual but by family and friends, or by staff if the older person has no family.

Choosing clothing

Some homes arrange trips into shopping centres so that older people can choose their own clothes. The local St John Ambulance, Red Cross, or Dial-A-Ride service often provide transport to enable people to make shopping trips. Some large stores have special open evenings for disabled people. Other large stores are willing to open for an extra hour and provide facilities for disabled and elderly people to shop after normal shopping hours. Some homes have companies come in with a selection of clothing and elderly people can select and try on clothes in the home. What arrangements has your home made to enable residents to choose their own clothing?

Advising disabled older people on choosing suitable clothing

Many disabled people have difficulty in dressing. Often choosing clothes that take account of the disability helps the older person to regain the ability to dress without help. Many women find front fastening dresses easier to put on. Dresses and blouses with wide sleeves are easier to put on than those with tight sleeves. Skirts and trousers with elasticated waistbands are easier to put on and more comfortable to wear than those with buttons at the waistband. A-line or full skirts are more comfortable to wear than straight skirts.

People who have difficulty doing up buttons and fasteners may find that:

- Large buttons are easier to fasten
- Zips are easier to do up than fasteners
- Elasticated trousers such as jogging pants may be more comfortable than other trousers
- Velcro can be used for fastenings on clothes

Helping people to help themselves

Many older people prefer to dress independently. Helping people to choose clothing that is easy to put on and fasten enables many individuals to remain independent. Many people find that aids help them retain their independence, such as the 'Helping Hand', a metal tool that can help an older person to put on stockings unaided. If you think that an older person might benefit from an aid, speak to senior staff about it.

Further reading

Jenkins, J. (1992) *The Clothes in Question*. Scutari Press, Harrow. This book gives advice and information on choosing, adapting and caring for people's clothes when they are living in homes.

Disabled Living Foundation (1994) *All Dressed Up*. Disabled Living Foundation, London. This book is full of practical advice and tips on choosing and adapting clothes. It also provides elderly people with advice on how to dress. There is a section on how to dress people who are unable to dress themselves.

Cosmetics

Some women living in nursing homes have been wearing cosmetics all their adult lives and feel naked without 'a touch of powder, rouge and lipstick'. Others prefer 'not to paint my face'. You should respect the individual's wishes. Some people find it difficult to apply make-up because of failing eyesight. Using a magnifying mirror can make it easier for the person to see more clearly. Some people may require help in putting on make-up, especially lipstick which can be difficult to apply if hands are not steady. People with sensitive skins can buy hypo-allergenic make-up that is less likely to cause allergies and skin reactions.

Summary

People of all ages enjoy looking and feeling good. Many older people living in homes require help with personal hygiene needs. The aim of care is to help or meet the hygiene needs of the older person. The rewards are enormous. Older people who are helped to regain or maintain independence feel in control of their lives and are happier and more fulfilled. People who are helped to look and feel good are less likely to become depressed and ill. You have the satisfaction of doing your job to the best of your ability.

Portfolio preparation

Some of the evidence you gather on this unit can be cross referenced to the moving and handling unit (Z7).

Your assessor must have evidence that you can meet the performance criteria for this unit. Before beginning this unit discuss assessment strategies with your assessor. Most of the evidence for this unit can be gained by direct observation of your work. You may be asked to provide the following types of evidence.

- Products. This might include your assessor looking at a person whom you have helped to bath, dress and groom.
- Witness testimony. This is a statement from a senior member of staff. It might be a statement detailing how you have met certain performance criteria.
- Written work. You might be asked to prepare a piece of work about how you enable older people to make real choices when helping them meet their hygiene needs. You might be asked to prepare a case study detailing how you meet an individual's hygiene needs.

Your assessor may also use other methods to help you gain evidence for this unit. These may include:

- Verbal questioning
- Written questions
- Watching you prepare equipment required to bedbath an individual. Watching you demonstrate how a hoist is used.

Further information

Health and Safety Executive (1992) Statutory Instrument no. 2793, the manual handling operations guidance regulations. Stationery Office, London.

References

Counsel & Care (1993) *The Right to Take Risks*. Counsel & Care, London.

Chapter 13

Promotion of Continence

Introduction

This chapter provides information on the option group A units Z11, Z11.1, Z11.2 and Z11.3 – 'enable clients to access and use toilet facilities'. It provides information on the normal functions of the bladder and bowel.

Information given in this chapter includes:

- Understanding elimination
- How ageing affects bladder function
- Enabling older people to use the toilet independently
- Dignity and privacy
- Health and safety
- Continence problems, including overactive bladder, stress and overflow incontinence
- How medicines, mobility and mental state affect continence
- Continence promotion – bladder re-training and timed voiding
- Incontinence pads
- Catheters and penile sheaths
- Bowel care
- Constipation
- Diarrhoea
- Stoma care
- Disposing of body waste

Understanding elimination

The kidneys produce urine and in doing so carry out three functions:

(1) Removing waste products from the blood
(2) Conserving water and salt
(3) Maintaining the balance of chemicals in the blood (electrolyte balance)

The amount of urine produced varies depending on the amount of fluid the person has consumed and the amount of fluid lost. On a very hot day, if the person does not drink extra fluid, the urine will become more concentrated. The kidneys concentrate the urine to maintain the balance of fluid within the body. If the person drinks a lot, more urine is produced. Many people notice that they pass more urine in cold weather; this is because less fluid is lost through sweating so urine production is increased to maintain the balance of fluid within the body. The average person drinking two litres of fluid each day will produce about 1500 +ml of urine each day. Most urine is formed when we are awake; at night, a hormone is produced which enables the kidneys to concentrate urine. This hormone is known as anti-diuretic hormone. The colour of urine varies according to how concentrated it is. Normally the urine passed first thing in the morning is darker because it is more concentrated. Urine is normally yellow or straw coloured.

Urine drains from the kidneys into the ureters (Fig. 13.1). It is then collected in the bladder. The bladder is a little like a balloon. It stretches in all directions to allow it to fill with urine and it contracts in all directions to empty. The bladder contains special nerves

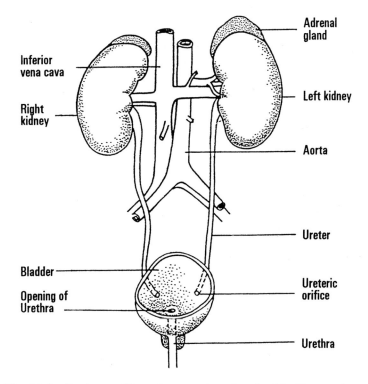

Fig. 13.1 Anatomy of the urinary system showing bladder, ureters and urethra.

known as stretch receptors. These send a message to the brain when the bladder is becoming full. The amount of urine the bladder holds varies; the male bladder can hold more than the female and some people have larger bladders than others. The urethra drains urine from the bladder.

How ageing affects the function of the kidneys and bladder

The kidneys work less efficiently in older people. They become less efficient at concentrating urine, so older people become dehydrated more easily than younger people. Older people usually produce more urine at night because of this. It is quite normal for an older person to have to get up once or twice in the night to pass urine. This is because the bladder becomes smaller in old age and less stretchy, and can hold less urine. When we pass urine a small amount is left in the bladder; this is known as residual urine. As people age and the bladder is less able to push urine out, the amount of urine left in the bladder increases.

Men have a gland known as the prostate gland, shown in Fig. 13.2. This enlarges with age and can make it more difficult for the

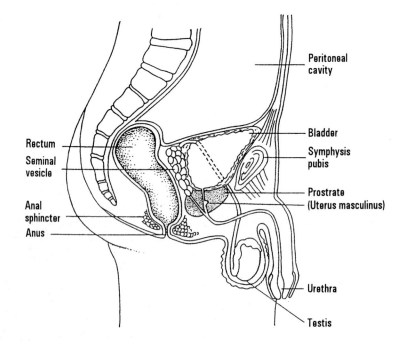

Fig. 13.2   Male genito-urinary tract.

bladder to empty completely. Women (Fig. 13.3) produce female hormones called oestrogen and progesterone. Hormone production is greatly reduced after the menopause and sometimes lack of oestrogen can lead to incontinence.

As people age the special nerves in the bladder (stretch receptors), which warn that the bladder is becoming full, become less sensitive. Adults are aware of the sensation of bladder fullness when the bladder is 50% full. The older person is not normally aware of the sensation of bladder fullness until the bladder is 90% full.

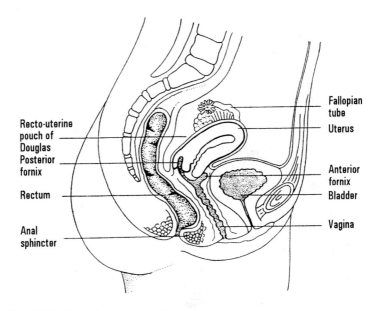

Recto-uterine pouch of Douglas

Posterior fornix

Rectum

Anal sphincter

Fallopian tube

Uterus

Anterior fornix

Bladder

Vagina

Fig. 13.3 Female genito-urinary tract.

Examining and testing urine

Normal urine is clear. Urine that is cloudy or thick or has bits floating in it should be saved and professional advice sought. Fresh urine does not smell. Urine which has been standing or which has been collecting in a catheter bag may smell because bacteria break down urine and produce ammonia. Urine should be golden or straw coloured. The first specimen of the day is usually darker. Dark urine is more concentrated than light urine and is normally a sign that the individual is not drinking enough. Some drugs and foods can cause the urine to change colour. Eating beetroot can produce red or pink urine. Some people who are prescribed the antibiotic nitofuridantoin produce turquoise urine.

If the urine looks abnormal in colour you should save the specimen and seek professional advice. Blood may cause the urine to appear red or pink. If you suspect that the urine contains blood, professional advice should be obtained immediately.

Urine is normally tested when an older person is admitted to the home. Testing urine enables staff to detect abnormalities. Urine is normally tested with a Multi-stick. This is a plastic strip that has a number of pads on it. Each pad has chemicals on it and changes colour when it is dipped in fresh urine and an abnormality is present. Urine is normally checked for a number of substances.

Blood
Blood in the urine can be caused by infection, kidney stones or other conditions.

Ketones
Ketones are substances produced when the body is burning up fat. This occurs if the person is diabetic and the diabetes is poorly controlled. Ketones are also present in the urine of people who are losing weight. The overweight person who is on a diet may have ketones in the urine. Undernourished people and people who have been vomiting (and are therefore not eating) may have ketones in their urine.

Glucose
Glucose is a form of sugar. It may be present in the urine of people who have diabetes.

Protein
Protein may be present in the urine of people who have kidney disease or who have a urine infection.

pH
pH indicates if the urine is acid or alkaline. Normally urine is slightly acid and has a pH of between five and seven. A pH above seven may indicate that the person has an infection. Vegetarians normally have a urine pH of above seven and this is normal for people who do not eat meat.

Specific gravity
Some urine testing sticks also measure the specific gravity. This enables staff to check how concentrated urine is. The normal specific gravity of urine is 1002 to 1030. A specific gravity of more than 1030 indicates that the urine is very concentrated.

Nitrite

Some sticks also test for nitrite. Nitrite is produced when an infection is present.

Urine test sticks will give inaccurate results if they are not stored properly. It is important to close the container tightly and not to remove the small packet which is in the bottle with the sticks. The packet contains crystals that prevent the sticks becoming damp and giving a false reading.

Faeces

Faeces contain waste products and food such as fibre that cannot be digested by the body. Faeces are normally brown and soft. Bile salts give faeces their brown colour. The normal stool is produced without straining. The amount of faeces produced varies according to how much fibre is eaten but between 80 and 200+g are produced each day. It normally takes three days for food to pass through the body. Bowel habits vary from individual to individual but research on large numbers of people shows that the normal range of bowel actions varies from three times per day to once every third day.

Some drugs can alter the appearance of faeces. Iron tablets cause the faeces to become black, sticky and look like tar. Some drugs can cause the individual to bleed either from the stomach or the bowel. Blood in faeces can also make them appear black and tar-like. If the individual bleeds from the lower bowel, blood can be seen clearly. If a resident passes faeces that appear abnormal, save the specimen or leave the toilet unflushed and obtain professional advice.

Enabling older people to use the toilet

Some older people living in homes will have difficulty walking. Often with help, encouragement, physiotherapy and walking aids they can regain the ability to walk to the toilet independently. Details on mobility are given in Chapter 9.

Some older people may have difficulty in identifying the toilets. If the toilets are in a corridor and all the doors look the same, it can be difficult to find the toilet. The older person with poor eyesight may be unable to read the small signs that say 'Toilet'. In some homes, all toilet doors have been painted a special colour, perhaps yellow, so that they stand out from all the other doors. In other homes, staff have made up large posters with pictures of toilets on them. Other homes have large signs saying 'Toilet' in letters six inches high. These measures help older people to find toilets quickly and enable them to use the toilet independently.

Some older men who have poor eyesight find it difficult to see the toilet. If the toilet and the floor are the same colour, a poorly sighted man can find this difficult. In some homes, a toilet seat in a contrasting colour such as black on a white toilet helps the person to see the toilet. This method works unless the male resident is in the habit of lifting the toilet seat, as many men do. In some homes, a coloured toilet cleanser is put in the cistern; each time the toilet is flushed, it refills with blue coloured water. The poorly sighted male resident can then aim for the blue water.

Some people who suffer from arthritis, especially arthritis of the hips and knees, can manage to sit on the toilet but find it difficult to get up because the seat is too low. Providing raised toilet seats that fit over the toilet can help people with arthritis to use the toilet independently.

Some people may find it difficult to pull down or adjust clothing without help. You can suggest clothing that is easier to remove and adjust. Trousers with elastic waistbands are easier to manage than those with zips and buttons. Some male residents find jogging pants comfortable, but these seldom have zips in the front. Placing a zip in the front helps many older men to use the toilet without help. Some men's trousers have short zips; if these are replaced with longer zips many male residents find it easier to use the toilet.

Female residents may have difficulty pulling up dresses or skirts that are tightly fitted around the legs and hips. Wearing skirts and dresses that are flared or have pleats makes it easier to hitch up clothing and use the toilet.

Male and female residents should be advised not to wear pants that are too tight. Tight pants are not only uncomfortable but are difficult to pull down. People who have difficulty dressing and undressing can be encouraged to practise. There are many ways of learning to dress and undress which take disability into account. Further details are given in *All Dressed Up*, the book mentioned under Further Reading in the Clothing section of Chapter 12.

Some older people become forgetful and may lose track of time. You can help by reminding forgetful residents to use the toilet. Reminding a person first thing in the morning, before meals and in the evening may help the older person to remain continent.

Dignity and privacy

Using the toilet is a private activity. Older people who are using the toilet should be able to do so without fearing that staff or other residents will burst in on them. Toilets should have locks and residents should be encouraged to lock the toilet door. If the older person is using a commode or bedpan, perhaps in a shared bedroom, the bed curtains should be drawn to protect the individual's privacy and dignity. Does your home have a policy on privacy and dignity?

Health and safety

Although the older person has the right to privacy and dignity when using the toilet, staff may need to enter the toilet in the case of an emergency. The individual may have fallen or collapsed and requires urgent help. Many homes have toilets that can be opened by staff in an emergency. Some homes have doors which open if the edge of a coin is inserted in a slot on the outside of the door, and turned. Other homes use a master key system; the key is placed in the outside of the lock and turned. Can the doors in your home be opened from the outside in an emergency?

Most toilets have vinyl floors. Many floors are made of special vinyl which is non-slip even when wet. There is a danger, though, that people will slip over if walking on a wet floor. If the toilet floor is wet it should be cleaned and dried at once to prevent falls occurring.

Most toilets have special rails that people can use to pull themselves up and hold onto when using the toilet. If these work loose, this should be reported at once. Normally the toilet should not be used until grab rails are made safe. If it is not possible to stop using the toilet, staff should accompany residents requiring help until repairs have been completed.

Toilets should have call bells fitted in case a person requires urgent help. Call bells should be within easy reach.

Assisting people to use toilets

Research shows that people are more likely to suffer from incontinence if they have to depend on someone else to take them to the toilet. It is easy to understand the reasons for this. An older person asks, 'Can you take me to the toilet please.' But the care assistant is busy laying the tables for lunch and says, 'Just a minute Mrs Johnston, I'll just finish laying the table.' The care assistant finishes laying the table and helps Mrs Johnston to the toilet. Mrs Johnston walks very slowly because she has had a stroke, her balance is poor and she uses a tripod. The toilet is some distance away. Just as they enter the toilet Mrs Johnston wets herself.

The section on the effects of ageing on the bladder at the beginning of this chapter explained how older people have less warning about the need to empty their bladders than younger people do. Mrs Johnston only became aware of the need to use the toilet when her bladder was almost full. She may have noticed that the staff were busy and waited until it seemed convenient; by then she was bursting to go. The well educated care assistant who is aware of how ageing and illness affect the bladder would have reacted differently. When Mrs Johnston asked to go to the toilet the care assistant would have come over at once and asked, 'Are you desperate or have we got time to walk there?' Mrs Johnston would have replied, 'No, I'm not desperate, we have plenty of time.' Because the care assistant responded promptly, Mrs Johnston had plenty of time to walk to the toilet. Had her need been more urgent, the care assistant could have wheeled her to the toilet and walked her back. The episode of incontinence would have been avoided.

If the older person is desperate to use the toilet but staff are encouraging the person to walk, wheeling her to the toilet and helping her to walk back will help the person to exercise and provide sensitive care.

If the person requires help to use the toilet, you should help the person to sit on the toilet, ensure that the individual can reach the call bell and offer to wait outside. The individual can call when she has finished. It is important to help the person to wash her hands after using the toilet. You should wash your hands every time you take an individual to the toilet. This is very important as it prevents the spread of infection.

Figure 13.4 shows a standing aid used to help a person use the the toilet.

Commodes

Commodes are sometimes used in homes. Often people who need to use the toilet at night are helped on and off commodes. Bedcurtains should be used at all times.

Bedpans

Bedpans are sometimes offered when the individual is in bed. It can be very difficult to sit comfortably on a bedpan and some people are unable to pass urine in them because they fear that the urine will splash on the bed. It is important to find out if the individual prefers to use a commode or a bedpan.

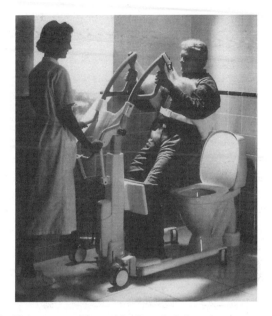

Fig. 13.4 Using a standing aid when helping a person to use the toilet.

How the bladder works

We are all born incontinent (Fig. 13.5) but learn to control our bladders as young children. When the bladder fills with urine it begins to contract and the urethra, which acts as a plug to hold urine in, relaxes. Urine is then forced out. When we develop control of our bladders, a signal is sent to our brain when the bladder is almost full. The brain then sends a signal back to the bladder telling it to hold on. This signals acts by stopping the bladder from contracting and tightening up the urethra. We then hold on until we can find a toilet, adjust our clothes and pass urine. This is demonstrated in Fig. 13.6. Normally people empty their bladders between four and eight times each day.

Continence problems

Incontinence is the inability to control bladder or bowels. Urinary incontinence, the inability to control the bladder, is much more common.

Most people feel that such a problem is shameful and are very embarrassed and upset by it. They fear that others may feel that they are dirty or lazy. Many older people who have

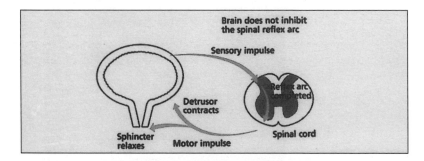

Fig. 13.5 A baby's bladder works by simple spinal reflex arc.

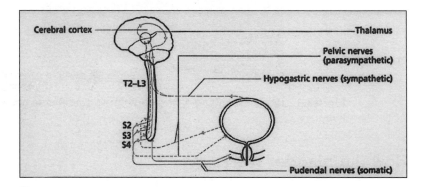

Fig. 13.6 Adult bladder control. Nerve pathways between the bladder, spine and micturition control centre. (Note: the nerves supplying the urethra are not shown in the diagram.)

problems controlling their bladders go to great lengths to conceal it. The older person living in a home may ask her family to bring in sanitary towels. She may use serviettes or toilet paper to line her pants. If her pants become wet she may wash them out and try to dry them on the radiator to prevent staff finding out.

Some staff working in homes, including some registered nurses, do not realise that many people who develop incontinence can be helped to become continent again. In some homes if a person becomes incontinent they are given pads and not treated. This is poor care. Incontinence is not a disease; it is a sign that something is wrong. It is often possible to discover and treat the problem causing the incontinence.

Continence assessments

Every person who has a continence problem should be seen and investigated. Professional staff who are qualified to carry out such investigations are:

- GPs
- District nurses
- Registered nurses

These staff may ask a nurse specially trained in helping people regain continence and in caring for incontinence. These nurses are known as continence advisers and have special training to help them work with people suffering from incontinence.

Causes of incontinence

There are many reasons why a person develops incontinence. Some of these are bladder problems but sometimes incontinence has other causes. The treatment given varies because the cause of incontinence is different in different people.

Overactive bladder

This is sometimes known as urgency or urge incontinence. The technical term for urge incontinence is bladder dysreflexia. You may notice:

- The person goes to the toilet very frequently and has to use the toilet more than twice each night
- The person has to rush to get to the toilet – sometimes just as she gets to the toilet she wets on the floor
- She may sometimes wet the bed a little at night.

Causes
The bladder muscles start to contract before the bladder is completely full. The individual is unable to stop the muscle contracting down and hold on. Urgency affects older men and women and is a very common problem. People who have had strokes or who suffer from Parkinson's disease may find urgency a problem. In many cases, the cause is still unknown. It is well known, though, that worry and nerves can make the bladder more likely to develop urgency. Some people find that when they are anxious they develop a headache or diarrhoea, while others find they keep needing to go to the toilet. If the older person is worried about wetting herself, this makes the situation worse.

Treatment

Urge incontinence is usually treated with bladder retraining. Details are given later in this chapter. In some cases drugs are also used.

Overflow incontinence

You may notice that:

- The person is always on the toilet
- The person is in there for ages
- The person has to strain to pass urine
- Urine is passed in little dribbles rather than a strong stream
- The person may dribble urine in between going to the toilet
- Only very small amounts of urine are passed although the person was desperate to go
- The individual complains that he or she has not been properly and the bladder still feels full

Causes

A blockage is preventing the bladder from emptying properly. The person can only pass small amounts of urine. The bladder is full and the person can only pass the small amount of urine, which is leaking or overflowing from the bladder. Overflow incontinence affects both men and women. It is commoner in men and can be caused by an enlarged prostate gland. Many people who have suffered from strokes or who have multiple sclerosis or motor neurone disease develop overflow incontinence. One of the commonest causes of overflow incontinence is constipation. A bowel full of faeces squeezes against the urethra and prevents urine draining.

Treatment

Treatment of overflow incontinence depends on the cause. Constipation is easily treated and effective bowel management will prevent it recurring. Men who are suffering from an enlarged prostate will be sent to see a consultant urologist who will decide on appropriate treatment. In some cases, catheters are used to drain urine. Further details on catheter care are given later in the chapter.

Stress incontinence

You may notice that:

- The bladder leaks when the individual coughs, sneezes or walks around

Causes

The bladder is supported by muscles known as the pelvic floor. These muscles can become weakened and support the bladder less effectively. Urine is held in the bladder and the urethra acts as a plug until it is convenient to pass urine. The urethra may become less effective in women after menopause due to a shortage of the hormone oestrogen. Stress incontinence normally affects women. Only men who have had surgery to the prostate gland may have problems with stress incontinence.

Treatment

Treatment will vary according to the cause. Weak muscles may be treated with pelvic floor exercises. If the muscles are very weak, surgery to repair the muscles and lift them back in place may be carried out. Many older women who have other health problems are not well enough to have surgery. A special ring (known as a ring pessary) may be inserted by a doctor or nurse specialist to hold up the womb if it is dropping down and pressing on the bladder. Sometimes these rings are coated with the female hormone oestrogen as this can help treat stress incontinence. These are usually changed by a doctor or nurse specialist every year. Sometimes a cream containing the hormone oestrogen is prescribed by the doctor. This is applied to the genital region and helps treat women who suffer from stress incontinence.

Other factors which cause incontinence

Many problems that cause incontinence are not bladder problems. Often the older person has been managing to control his or her bladder until a change in circumstances tips the individual over the edge into incontinence. Many things can cause incontinence, including the attitude of staff. The commonest reasons older people develop continence problems are given below.

Moving to a new place

Often when the older person is to be admitted to the home, staff ask if the person has a continence problem. The answer is often no, yet when the person arrives at the home she is incontinent. Leaving his or her own home where a person has lived for many years and entering a residential or nursing home is a stressful experience. The older person is usually admitted from hospital and may dread entering the home. She may have been transferred from an acute ward to an elderly care ward and then finally to the home. This makes older people anxious and worried. Stress and worry can affect the bladder and cause incontinence. Helping the person settle into the home, making her feel welcome and providing sensitive care can help clear up the incontinence quickly. Further details are given in Chapters 7 and 8.

Medicines

Medicines can cause incontinence. They can act in a number of ways, either working directly on the bladder or affecting the person's general health.

Diuretics are often referred to as water tablets. Diuretics stimulate the kidneys and increase the amount of urine produced. Diuretics are given to treat heart failure, to lower blood pressure or to treat swollen legs. There are many different types of diuretics. Some act slowly and gently, causing a little more urine to be produced throughout the day. Others have a more drastic action and cause the kidneys to produce large amounts of urine for a few hours. Diuretics are usually given in the morning. This can cause problems if the older person requires help to go to the toilet as staff are busiest in the morning, and a delay in responding to the person's request for help can lead to incontinence.

In some homes, older people have sleeping tablets every night. Sleeping tablets cause people to be less alert and drowsier, not just at night but also during the day. They can lead to incontinence. Some older people are anxious and upset when they enter homes. Some are prescribed sedatives and these can cause the person to become less alert and to become incontinent.

Other medicines can also cause incontinence. A continence assessment by a trained professional will include checking the person's medication. If medication is causing incontinence this may be discontinued or changed by the person's doctor.

Difficulty with walking

The older person who is unable to use the toilet without help is more likely to suffer from incontinence. Chapter 7 gives details of how you can help older people regain independence. Chapter 9 gives information on helping the older person to move. It is important to respond promptly to calls for help to use the toilet.

Confusion

The person who is confused or forgetful may have problems remembering to go to the toilet. Reminding the person to go to the toilet at set times often helps to prevent incontinence.

Infection

A bladder infection causes the bladder to become more irritable. The person who has a bladder infection usually needs to go to the toilet frequently and pass small amounts of urine. Bladder infections can cause the individual to become confused and this can lead to incontinence.

Often confusion is one of the first signs of a chest infection in elderly people. Older people can become very ill if they are suffering from a chest infection. The individual may be unable to walk to the toilet and because of confusion may be unable to ask for the toilet. Coughing can lead to stress incontinence. Fortunately, the incontinence normally vanishes when the person recovers from the infection.

How you can help

Don't take incontinence for granted. If an older person is developing bladder problems seek professional advice. A continence assessment will usually be carried out to find out why the person has become incontinent. You may be asked to help by keeping a fluid balance chart. This involves keeping a record of everything a person drinks and all urine passed. The fluid chart is normally recorded for a week. The registered nurse or continence adviser may then ask for a bladder chart to be used. A copy is shown in Fig. 13.7.

Each time the person passes urine in the toilet the left hand side of the chart is ticked. Each time the person is wet, the right hand side of the chart is ticked. The chart is used to monitor the person's progress and to help decide on further treatment. This will vary from person to person and will depend on the nature of the problem.

Bladder retraining

Bladder retraining is used to help people who suffer from urgency and have overactive bladders to regain control of the bladder. The bladder chart enables staff to see how often the person can hold on between visits to the toilet. The individual is encouraged to hold on for an extra 15 minutes between each visit to the toilet. Every three days the time between visits is increased by 15 minutes. Gradually the bladder stretches and is able to hold more urine. The person learns to control bladder contractions. Eventually the older person should be able to visit the toilet every two or three hours. Sometimes drugs are given to help increase the amount of urine the bladder can hold and dampen down bladder contractions. These drugs are known as anticholinergics.

BLADDER CHART

Week commencing: Name:

Please tick in the **plain** column each time you pass urine

Please tick in the **shaded** column each time you are wet

Special instructions:

	Monday	Tuesday	Wednesday	Thursday	Friday	Saturday	Sunday
Midnight							
1am							
2							
3							
4							
5							
6							
7							
8							
9							
10							
11							
Noon							
1pm							
2							
3							
4							
5							
6							
7							
8							
9							
10							
11							
Totals							

BLADDER TRAINING PROGRAMME

In order to bring your bladder problem under control, you must learn to stretch your bladder. You can do this by trying to hold on as long as possible before passing water. Do not restrict your fluid intake. You should drink no more or less than you normally do.

On the back of this sheet is a bladder chart to help you monitor your progress – fill this in **every time you pass urine normally** and **every time you are wet.**

❑ Please a tick in the shaded column to the nearest hour when you leak urine, place a tick in the **plain** column when you pass urine normally.

❑ When you get the feeling that you want to pass urine **try to hold on for as long as possible.**

❑ At first this will be difficult, but as you persevere it will become easier.

❑ If you wake up at night with a full bladder it is best to go and empty it straight away, as holding on will only keep you awake.

❑ Sitting on a hard seat may help you to hold your water.

❑ Your doctor may have prescribed tablets to help you hold your water. Take these regularly as directed.

❑ You should aim to gradually reduce the frequency with which you pass urine to 5 or 6 times in 24 hours.

REMEMBER

You are attempting to stretch your bladder. Although you may find this difficult at first, with practice it will get easier. If you persevere, you will be surprised at what you can achieve.

Fig. 13.7 Bladder chart.

Timed voiding

People who are confused or forgetful often forget to go to the toilet or do not understand the messages they receive to tell them their bladder is full up. The bladder chart enables staff to discover the times the person is normally wet. The person is taken to the toilet before the time of incontinence and encouraged to use the toilet. Using this method, it is possible to help about two-thirds of all confused people regain continence. Unfortunately about one-third do not have a regular pattern of passing urine and timed toileting is hit and miss.

Caring for people who are incontinent

Some people cannot be helped to regain continence. Incontinence may be caused by either a physical problem such as motor neurone disease or an enlarged prostate, or a mental problem such as dementia. The aim of care is to collect the urine, prevent the person becoming smelly, sore or wet, protect the skin and ensure that the person's dignity is maintained at all times.

Incontinence pads

Incontinence pads are used to collect urine. They normally have a plastic backing and are filled with cellulose pulp (Fig. 13.8). The superabsorbent pads contain granules that swell up and form a gel when wet. This gel locks the urine into the pad and helps keep the person's skin dry. Many pads have a liner that draws urine away from the skin.

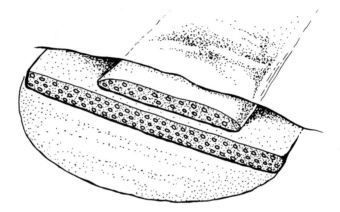

Fig. 13.8   Incontinence pad.

Some pads have a wetness indicator in the plastic outer covering of the pad. The wetness indicator changes colour when the pad needs changing. If the person has been incontinent of faeces, the pad should be changed immediately to maintain comfort and prevent skin problems.

Pads work more effectively and are less likely to leak if they are fitted closely to the body. Most pad manufacturers recommend that the person wears a pair of specially designed briefs made of nylon to hold the pad in place (Figs 13.9 and 13.10).

How often should pads be changed?

This will vary from person to person and will depend on the amount of urine produced. Pads may be changed every two to four hours. Pads should not be left unchanged for longer than four hours or skin problems can occur. Many pads now have a wetness

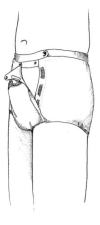
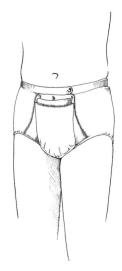

(a)

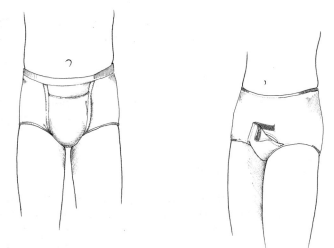

(b)

Fig. 13.9 Marsupial pants are washable; a pad is inserted into a plastic pouch and changed when wet: (a) male marsupial pants; (b) female marsupial pants.

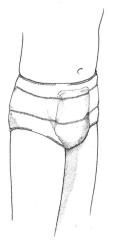

Fig. 13.10 An incontinence pad held in position by specially designed pants.

indicator to alert staff when pads need changing. Details on caring for the skin of incontinent people are given in Chapter 12.

Dribble pads

These are small pads which fit over the penis and collect small drips or dribbles. Their use can preserve dignity, protect clothing and prevent odour.

Special underwear

It is now possible to buy pants with a built-in washable incontinence pad. These are available for men and women. They come in a range of sizes and a variety of styles. These small pads can absorb up to 80 ml of urine. Some female residents who suffer from slight stress incontinence prefer these to a pad. Some male residents who leak small amounts of urine find pants more normal and acceptable than dribble pads. The pants are, of course, named and are the personal underwear of that particular person. It is important not to use fabric conditioner on these pants as it prevents them absorbing urine.

Re-usable incontinence pads

Re-usable incontinence pads are now available. These are provided to individual residents, named, laundered and returned to the individual. They are available in a range of sizes and absorbencies. Re-usable pads increase demands on the laundry. They are not commonly used within nursing homes.

Obtaining incontinence pads

At the moment people who suffer from incontinence and who are cared for in residential homes are issued with pads by the local NHS trust. If you work in a home run by social services, these pads are delivered to the home. In most areas staff working in private residential homes collect the pads once a week. In nursing homes, the home is responsible for buying the pads.

Disposing of incontinence pads

Used incontinence pads cannot be disposed of with normal household waste. Homes have a duty under the Environmental Protection Act 1990 to ensure that pads are disposed of properly. Homes use different systems to dispose of incontinence pads. Some homes use a macerator; the pads are placed in the macerator and are reduced to a pulp and washed away into the drain. Other homes use a yellow bag system. All body waste, which is to be taken away from the home and disposed of, should be collected in a yellow plastic bag. These bags are stored in special sack holders in the sluice room. The bags are either collected by the local council or by a private firm. Homes are charged for each sack of clinical waste removed. The waste is then incinerated at high temperature.

Penile sheaths

Penile sheaths look like condoms (Fig. 13.11). They are attached to the penis using either a special adhesive or a strap; the lower end has an outlet, which is connected to a catheter bag. The bag is strapped to the leg. Urine drains from the penis into the catheter bag. Some men find this convenient and comfortable, while others do not. Penile sheaths should be removed daily. Particular care must be taken to enable the person to maintain personal hygiene. Sheaths can cause soreness and this can lead to infection. If the person's skin appears red or sore, seek professional help. It is important to seek professional advice if the person finds a penile sheath uncomfortable or would prefer to use a different method to contain incontinence.

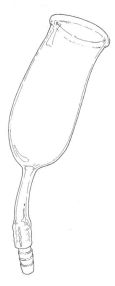

Fig. 13.11   Urinary sheath.

Catheters

Catheters are inserted through the urethra and into the bladder. They are held in place by a balloon, which is filled with sterile water. Urine is drained from the bladder by the catheter and is collected in a catheter bag. Professional staff should avoid using catheters simply to contain incontinence. They are used only when no other method of controlling incontinence will be effective. People who suffer from overflow incontinence, who have failed to respond to treatment, or who are too frail for surgery may have their incontinence managed by using a catheter. People who have a catheter can develop problems. These include blockage, leaking, pain and infection. If problems occur, seek professional advice.

Catheter bags

Urine drains from the catheter into a catheter bag (Fig. 13.12a). There are two different types of catheter bag, for night and day use. Night drainage bags are large bags. They are supported on stands which are suspended on the bed or sit on the floor beside the bed. Leg bags are worn during the day (Fig. 13.12b). These are strapped to the person's leg and hidden by either a skirt or trousers. It is important to support catheter bags by using either a stand or strapping them to the leg. Catheter bags fill with urine and can become very heavy. If the bag is not supported the weight of

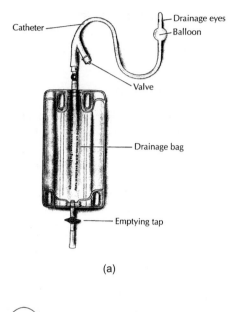

(a)

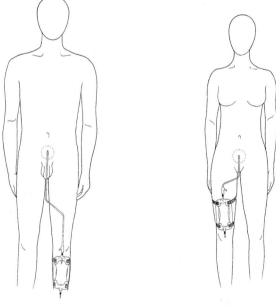

(b)

Fig. 13.12 (a) Catheter and drainage bag; (b) catheter and leg bag.

urine can pull the catheter and cause the neck of the bladder, where the balloon sits, to become bruised and swollen. This can cause pain and bleeding.

Emptying catheter bags

Catheter bags should be emptied every four hours. If the person is passing a lot of urine, you may need to empty the bag more frequently. The bag should be emptied before it is completely full to avoid pulling on the delicate tissues at the neck of the bladder. Hands are washed and disposable gloves put on. Urine should be drained into a jug which has been sterilised in the bedpan washer. The urine is then tipped down the bedpan washer and the jug re-sterilised. Gloves should be removed and hands washed.

How often should catheter bags be changed?

The Department of Health recommends that catheter bags are changed twice each week. It can be difficult for staff to keep track of when a catheter bag was last changed as one person may change the bag before going off duty for a few days. The person returning from days off may be unaware of this and may change the bag again. In some homes when a bag is changed the date of the change is written discreetly on the inner side of the bag with a marking pen, as well as recorded on the care plan.

Bowel function

The large bowel is known as the colon. It absorbs water and salts, and the remaining waste product, faeces, is passed into the rectum. When we eat, the contents of the bowel move into the rectum. We then feel that the rectum is full and we need to open our bowels. This is known as the gastrocolic reflex. This reflex is strongest after breakfast.

Constipation

Constipation can occur if a person does not go to the toilet when the rectum is full. The person may, because of a loss of sensation, be unaware of the need to go to the toilet. The person may be reluctant to open their bowels. This may be because there is little privacy in the home or the person may feel rushed. The person may find opening the bowels is painful because of diseases such as haemorrhoid.

Constipation can also occur if the person's diet does not have enough fibre. Advice on a high fibre diet is given in Chapter 6. If the person is not drinking enough fluid, this can also lead to constipation. People who are not active and who do not walk about are more likely to suffer from constipation. Helping and encouraging the older person to walk will often help prevent constipation.

If the older person remains constipated despite eating a high fibre diet, drinking enough fluid and moving around, seek professional advice. The nurse, doctor or continence adviser will investigate the reasons for constipation and plan treatment. Investigation will include checking the medication that the older person is taking. Some medication can cause constipation.

Diarrhoea

Diarrhoea is the frequent passage of loose or liquid stools. The commonest causes of diarrhoea are laxatives, antibiotics, food poisoning and faecal impaction.

Laxatives
Laxatives can be given to treat constipation, but it can be extremely difficult to calculate the dose required to enable an individual to have a normal bowel action. If the older person is eating a diet high in fibre, is drinking sufficient fluids and is encouraged to move around, laxatives will seldom be required.

Antibiotics
Antibiotics given to treat an infection can often cause diarrhoea. The most effective way of preventing infection and reducing antibiotic use is careful handwashing.

Food poisoning
Food poisoning can cause diarrhoea. Staff who do not carefully wash their hands after attending to each resident, and do not maintain resident hygiene and carefully dispose of body fluids according to the home's policy, can contribute to an outbreak of diarrhoea within the home.

Constipation
Constipation can also lead to diarrhoea. Hard, dried faeces build up in the rectum and cannot be passed. Further faeces gather behind this and can leak around the blockage. Although it appears that the person has diarrhoea, severe constipation is the real problem.

Caring for the person with diarrhoea

If the older person develops diarrhoea, seek professional advice. Treatment will depend on the cause of the diarrhoea. The older person may no longer require laxatives if they are causing the problem. It may be possible for the doctor to change the antibiotic the person is taking if this is causing the diarrhoea. The person with food poisoning may require treatment if the diarrhoea is severe. The person with severe constipation will require treatment to clear the bowel.

It is important to encourage people with diarrhoea to drink plenty of fluids as extra fluid is being lost through the faeces and this must be replaced. The person who has diarrhoea may need assistance to get to the toilet in time. In some cases, a commode by the bed will be required. The person's privacy and dignity should be maintained at all times and air fresheners should be used to ensure the room does not smell, as this could embarrass the individual.

Soiled linen

Every home should have a policy for dealing with soiled linen. Normally it is placed in red plastic bags with an alginate strip. This is taken to the laundry where it is laundered separately from all other linen. The bag is normally placed in the washing machine and placed on sluice cycle. The alginate strip then dissolves and the bag opens. The laundry is rinsed and the bag is then disposed of. The linen is then washed normally.

Stoma care

A stoma is a piece of bowel that has been brought to the surface of the abdomen (Fig. 13.13). The stoma normally looks pink or red. The stoma takes the place of the anus and faeces pass through the stoma. The person with a stoma has no control over when the faeces will come out and must wear a bag to collect faeces (Fig. 13.14). The stoma is made from the large bowel. The large bowel absorbs water so the stool of a person with a colostomy will resemble a normal stool. The person with a colostomy uses a closed bag. When the person has passed a stool the bag is removed and replaced with a new bag.

A person who has a stoma formed from the small intestine (known as an ileostomy) will pass a liquid stool. The amount of stool will be greater and people who have ileostomies will need to drink extra fluid because of this. People who have ileostomies normally wear a drainage bag and the stool is drained into a jug.

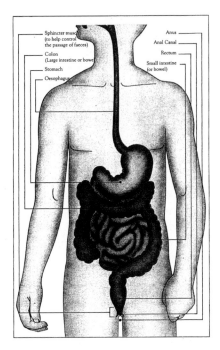

(a)

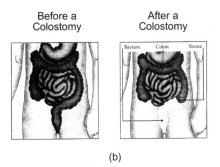

Before a
Colostomy

After a
Colostomy

(b)

Fig. 13.13 (a) Normal digestive system; (b) intestines before and after a colostomy.

Disposing of body waste

If the older person has a stoma, there are normally two different methods of disposing of the body waste. All stoma bags come complete with a small bag with two handles. The bag is designed to hold the stoma bag and then tie up. This sealed bag is then placed in the yellow clinical waste container. In some homes faeces are tipped out of the bag and disposed of in the bedpan

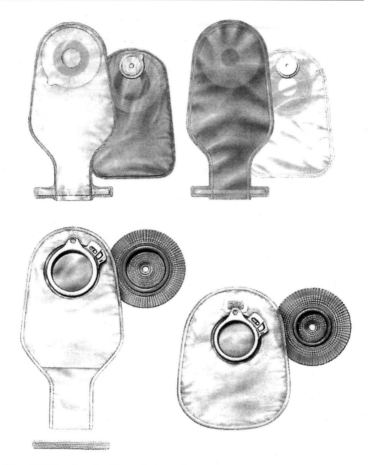

Fig. 13.14   A selection of stoma bags.

washer. The empty bag is then placed in a bag, sealed and placed in the yellow clinical waste bag.

If the older person has an ileostomy, the faecal fluid is normally drained into a special jug that is usually named, e.g. Mrs Jones, stomal effluent only. The fluid is disposed of in the bedpan washer. Figure 13.15 shows a typical bedpan washer. The jug is then re-sterilised for future use. This jug is kept separate from others and is never used to drain urine from catheter bags.

Summary

Enabling and helping the older person to use the toilet can prevent incontinence. Investigation and treatment can help many older people regain continence. Some older people are unable to regain

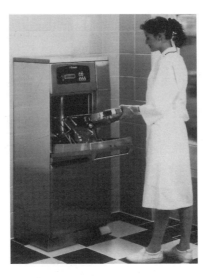

Fig. 13.15   A bedpan washer.

continence and it is important that you help to contain incontinence and help prevent skin problems. Older people may feel embarrassed about requiring help to use the toilet or to deal with incontinence. Great sensitivity is required and the carer's attitude is of prime importance in helping older people accept help while maintaining self-esteem.

Portfolio preparation

Collecting evidence for this unit causes great problems for some assessors and students. There are reports of registered nurse assessors and two members of staff assisting residents to the toilet. Some assessors feel that they cannot help a resident and assess at the same time. If the assessor is a registered nurse who normally works in the home, I personally do not feel that assessing and assisting are inappropriate.

Your assessor must have evidence that you can meet the performance criteria for this unit. Before beginning this unit discuss assessment strategies with your assessor. Sensitive assessors who normally work in the home as a member of staff can help you gain most of the evidence for this unit by direct observation of your work. However, if the assessor is not normally involved in direct care within the home then you may have to use simulations to gain some of the evidence. You may be asked to provide the following types of evidence:

- Products.
- Witness testimony. This is a statement from a senior member of staff. It might be a statement detailing how you have met certain performance criteria.
- Written work. You might be asked to prepare a piece of work about how you enable a resident to maintain dignity when he or she relies on staff to help use the toilet. You might be asked to reflect on an incident when you felt the person's dignity was compromised, and the lessons you learnt.

Assessment strategies for this unit will vary depending on the availability of a work based assessor. Your assessor may also use other methods to help you gain evidence for this unit. These may include:

- Verbal questioning
- Written questions
- Watching you disinfect a bedpan after use, and watching you prepare a commode for use

Simulations may be used to help gain evidence if it cannot be gained by direct observation

Telephone help-lines

A number of organisations and companies who supply incontinence products have a telephone service. People suffering from incontinence, care assistants or registered nurses can telephone and ask for advice.

The Bard help-line is open from 12.30PM–4.30PM Monday to Friday. Tel. 0800 591 783.

Coloplast Service help-line is open from 9AM–5PM Monday to Friday. Tel. 0800 22 06 22.

Hollister Incare help-line is open from 9AM–5PM Monday to Friday. Tel. 0800 521 377.

The incontinence information help-line is run by a charity and offers advice and help. The lines are open from 2PM–7PM. Tel. 0191 0050.

Further information

The Alzheimer's Disease Society
158–160 Balham High Road
London SW12 9BN
Tel. 020 8675 6557
This society produces a booklet and a leaflet on caring for people
with dementia who have continence problems. Send a large SAE,
with two first class stamps.

The Continence Foundation
307 Hatton Square
16 Baldwin Gardens
London EC1N 7RJ
Tel. 020 7404 6875
The Continence Foundation produces a great deal of information
on continence care, including a booklet on maintaining bowel
control.

The British Colostomy Association
15 Station Road
Reading RG1 1LG
Tel. 0118 939 1537
Helpline 0800 328 4257
This charity offers information and advice to people who have
colostomies, and produces a number of useful leaflets. It also
provides a network of volunteers who are themselves colosto-
mists. The volunteers will visit and provide advice and support to
residents who have colostomies.

Further reading

There are a number of books dealing with the subject of continence promotion and the management of incontinence. The
books listed are suitable for care assistants. You may be able to
obtain these either from the library of the college where you are
studying or from the local library.

Castledean, C.M. & Duffin, H. (1991) *Staying Dry: Advice for
Sufferers of Incontinence*. Quay Publishing, 11 Victoria
Wharf, St George's Quay, Lancaster LA1 1GA. This book is
aimed at people who suffer from incontinence. It is simple and
easy to understand and care assistants will find it useful.

Fader, M. & Norton C. (1994) *Caring for Continence*. Hawker
Publications Ltd, 13 Park House, 140 Battersea Park Road,

London SW11 4NB. This book has been written specially for care assistants studying at NVQ levels 2 and 3.

Norton, C. (1996) *Nursing for Continence*, 2nd edn. Beaconsfield Publishers Ltd, 20 Chiltern Hills Road, Beaconsfield, Buckinghamshire HP9 1PL. This is a more detailed book that has been written for the registered nurse with an interest in continence care. If you wish to study the subject in greater depth, this is the best book to start with. Although it is written for registered nurses, it is easy to read and a full explanation of all terms is given.

Glossary

Anaemia: A reduction in the number of red cells or the amount of haemoglobin (the substance in red blood cells which carries oxygen); causes of anaemia include poor diet and bleeding.

Alzheimer's disease: A progressive disorder of the brain. It causes total disintegration of the personality and eventually the person loses the ability to reason and to carry out the activities of daily living. There is no known cure for this terminal disease.

Angina: Lack of oxygen to the heart muscle caused by narrowing or blockage of the arteries supplying the heart with blood.

Anomia: Difficulty in finding words.

Aphasia: Inability to speak.

Arthritis: Pain, stiffness and sometimes inflammation of one or more joints.

Asthma: Narrowing of the bronchial tubes which allow air into the lungs. Caused by allergies including medication, dust and pollen. Treated with tablets and inhalers which help the bronchial tubes to relax and open, allowing air to pass freely into the lungs.

Bladder dysreflexia: *See* overactive bladder.

Capillaries: Small blood vessels that carry oxygen and glucose to the tissues.

Cataract: The lens of the eye, which we look through in order to see clearly, becomes white, cloudy and milky in appearance. This affects the vision and can, depending on how severe it is, lead to visual problems or blindness. Treatment is surgical. The cataract is removed and usually a contact lens is inserted into the eye to replace the lens which has been removed.

Catheter (urinary): A tube which passes from the urethra to the bladder and is used to drain urine.

Cellulitis: Inflammation of tissue. This term is normally used to refer to an inflammation of the skin.

Cerebrovascular accident: A medical term for a stroke.

Colles' fracture: A fracture of the wrist.

Constipation: No bowel action for three days or more or passing very hard dry stools which may resemble rabbit droppings.

Decubitus ulcer: Medical term used for pressure sore.

Deep vein thrombosis: A clot which forms in either the deep veins of the legs or pelvis. This clot can break off and travel around the body until it becomes stuck in an artery. This is known as a pulmonary embolus. People who are immobile are at risk of developing a deep vein thrombosis.

Dementia: *See* Alzheimer's disease and multi-infarct dementia.

Diabetes: This is known as diabetes mellitus (sweet diabetes) because the urine contains sugar. This condition was first described by the ancient Greeks who diagnosed it by tasting the urine. The body is unable to use glucose (sugar) because of absence or shortage of insulin. Treatment is either by diet, so that the overweight diabetic loses weight and there is enough insulin to go round, or tablets to make the body produce more insulin, or insulin injections. Untreated diabetes leads to high levels of sugar in the blood. These high sugar levels can cause kidney damage, blindness and circulation problems.

Dysarthria: Difficulty in forming and articulating words.

Dysphasia: Difficulty in speaking or understanding words. *See* expressive dysphasia and receptive dysphasia.

Elder abuse: Mistreatment of an older person. It can be a single act or a long-term pattern of abuse.

Electrolytes: Balance of chemicals in the blood. These can become unbalanced because of disease, medication or poor diet.

Expressive dysphasia: General difficulty in expressing what a person wishes to say.

Fracture: A broken bone.

Gastrostomy: An opening from the stomach to the skin. This is created by a surgeon to enable nursing staff to feed people who are unable to swallow. A tube is placed into this opening and special liquid feeds are given.

Glaucoma: An eye condition which causes the pressure within the eye to become raised. There are a number of different types of glaucoma. Glaucoma can be treated medically or surgically. Untreated glaucoma can cause blindness.

Hemianopia: loss of sight in half the visual field. This means that the person has 'blind spots' and visual difficulties.

Hemiplegia: Paralysis of one side of the body usually as the result of a stroke or injury to the brain.

Incontinence: The inability to 'hold on' to urine or faeces until a suitable place can be found to empty the bladder or bowel.

Intravenous infusion: This is commonly known as a 'drip'. Sterile fluid is given slowly into a vein.

Ketones: Substances which are produced within the body and removed in the urine when the body is burning fat. Seen in poorly controlled diabetics, people who have been vomiting and in starvation.

Motor neurone disease: A progressive degenerative condition. The neurones (nerve cells) degenerate leading to paralysis and eventually death. There is no known cure.

Multi-infarct dementia: Interruption of the blood supply to the brain by a small clot, causing tissue death. These small clots cause brain tissue to die and the person loses the ability to reason and function if treatment is not effective. Treatment, such as control of high blood pressure and giving a small dose of aspirin, aims to prevent clots forming in the circulation of the brain.

Nasogastric tube: A tube which goes down the nose and into the stomach. It is used to give fluids directly into the stomach when a person is unable to swallow, perhaps because of a stroke or motor neurone disease.

Osteo-arthritis: Arthritis of the hands, knees, hips and big toes.

Osteoporosis: Thinning and weakening of the bones which makes them fracture more easily.

Overactive bladder: The bladder muscle contracts before it is completely full. The person passes small amounts of urine frequently and may find it difficult to hold on until the toilet can be reached. This can be caused by strokes or Parkinson's disease.

Overflow incontinence: Difficulty in emptying the bladder completely caused by a blockage. Constipation, Parkinson's disease and an enlarged prostate are some of the causes of overflow incontinence.

Parkinson's disease: A brain disorder caused by a reduction of a chemical, called dopamine, in the brain. It is a progressive disease and eventually the person loses the ability to carry out the activities of daily living. It causes difficulty in moving and speaking. In the early stages medication helps control symptoms.

Penile sheath: A condom-like device which fits over the penis and drains urine into a catheter bag.

Pressure sore: An area of tissue which has died because unrelieved pressure has caused the circulation to the tissue to be cut off. Pressure sores can affect skin, fat, muscle and bone, depending on the severity.

Pulmonary embolus: A clot which forms in the deep veins of the leg or pelvic veins, breaks off and travels to the heart. It can cause death by blocking a heart valve or the pulmonary artery. A smaller clot can damage lung tissue.

Receptive dysphasia: Difficulty or inability to make sense of messages received by speech.

Rheumatoid arthritis: An inflammatory disease of the joints. The synovial tissue that covers the joints becomes inflamed.

This causes the affected joints to become hot, swollen and painful.

Shearing forces: Damage to the capillary circulation caused by dragging or friction. The damage caused can lead to pressure sores developing.

Specific gravity: A way of checking how concentrated urine is. This enables staff to discover if a person is not having enough fluid.

Stoma: A stoma is an opening from the inside of the body to the outside. A colostomy is an opening created by a surgeon from the large bowel (colon) to the surface of the abdomen. An ileostomy is an opening from the small bowel (ileum) to the surface of the abdomen. Body waste which comes out of these stomas is collected in a bag.

Stress incontinence: A leak of urine on moving, coughing or sneezing. Caused by weakness of the muscles in the pelvic floor.

Stroke: An interruption of the blood supply to the brain caused by either bleeding or a clot. This leads to an area of tissue death and also bruising to brain tissue.

Synovial fluid: A thick fluid that surrounds the end of the bone and the cartilage.

Urethra: The tube that enables the bladder to discharge urine.

Index